LOOK 15 YEARS YOUNGER

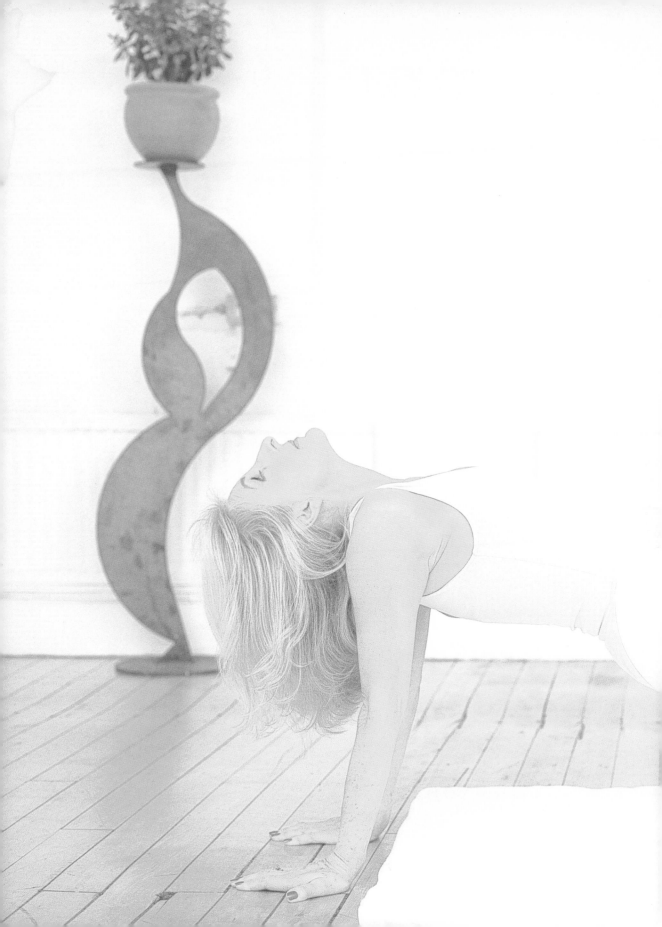

LOOK 15 YEARS YOUNGER

Barbara Currie

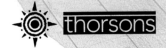
thorsons

To my wonderful family: my mother Babs, my husband Gordon, my daughter Lysanne, my son Mark, my daughter-in-law Rachel and my brother Richard and his family. I am most grateful to you all for your kindness and unconditional love and support.

Thorsons
An imprint of HarperCollins*Publishers*
77–85 Fulham Palace Road,
Hammersmith, London W6 8JB

The website address is: www.thorsonselement.com

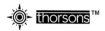

and *Thorsons* are trademarks of
HarperCollins*Publishers* Limited

First published by Thorsons 2003

10 9 8 7 6 5 4 3 2 1

Photography by Guy Hearn

A catalogue record of this book
is available from the British Library

ISBN 0 00 715540 9

Printed and bound in Great Britain by
Scotprint, Haddington, East Lothian

Not all exercises are suitable for everyone. To reduce the risk to
you, please consult your doctor before beginning this exercise
programme. The instructions and advice presented are in no way
intended as a substitute for medical guidance. The writer and
publishers of this book do not accept any responsibility for any
injury or accident as a result of following this exercise programme.

contents

Acknowledgements

I am most grateful to my agent Sue Ayton and my literary agent, Michael Alcock, for their enthusiasm, help and support. Very many thanks to Wanda Whiteley for her inspiration and encouragement and for making this book possible. Thank you to Claire Dunn for your help and kindness during the photo shoot and throughout this project. My thanks go to Simon Gerratt and Barbara Vesey for their thoughtfulness, hard work and tremendous care in editing my script. Many thanks to Guy Hearn for his beautiful photography and to Sallyann Sexton for taking so much care over hair and makeup for both my students and me. A big thank you to Polly Zabari for typing my initial script with such speed and enthusiasm.

I am so grateful to Natasha Fidler for the beautiful design of this book and to Sonia Dobie for the lovely cover. Thank you Maureen Barrymore for the excellent cover photograph. I would also like to thank my students Nicky Bell, Rachel Thompson, Julie Brittle, Liz Richardson and Lisa Smart for posing so beautifully for the photographs and to Joanne Cassidy who helped us all during the photoshoot with incredible care and patience. I am so grateful to many of my students who have sent me their own inspirational quotes that have been included in this book.

Thank you. Thank you to you all.

Introduction

Since the beginning of time, man has searched for that magical something to give him eternal youth.

Today this searching is at an all-time high, with billions being spent on miracle 'get young' face creams, neck creams, eye creams, cosmetic surgery, botox injections, collagen implants and facials, all with the ultimate quest of looking and feeling younger and halting the advance of the years.

But why do we want to be and look younger? When we were young, did we appreciate it? Didn't we curse the spots and pimples, the lack of self-esteem, the school exams, relationship problems, etc? We had unlined skin, but did we appreciate that? Didn't we cover it with make-up and try to look years older than we were? So what is it that we yearn for about youth? Do we really want to put the clock back and go through all those years again? – I doubt it!

George Bernard Shaw once said, 'Youth is wasted on the young?' Isn't what we are searching for something quite, quite different? Wouldn't we rather keep our present age but have the radiance, amazing energy, excitement, flexibility and agility of youth? Wouldn't we like to get rid of the sagging muscles, aches and pains, excess weight, diminished eyesight and hearing and memory loss and replace it with a toned, firm and beautiful body, amazing energy, glowing, unwrinkled skin and improved memory, eyesight and hearing? Wouldn't we like to be able to stay calm under stress, sleep really well at night and wake with that good-to-be-alive feeling and keep making new goals and planning new ventures regardless of our age?

If you are answering 'yes' to any of the above, then **yoga is for you**. I became a yoga addict at my very first yoga class over 30 years ago. I was stiff, tired, tense and out of sorts when I enrolled to try yoga for the very first time, but the sight of my teacher, then in her late fifties, will stay in my memory for ever. She was perfectly toned and, as she stood to demonstrate posture after posture, she did it with the flexibility, ease – and body shape – of an 18 year old.

She didn't look tired or tense, but radiated a wonderful zest for life that was contagious and I left my first class walking taller and feeling better than I had felt for ages.

As I continued to learn yoga, from time to time I received some jolts or wake-up calls as ancient legends and parables were recited to us teaching us age-old truths. This is one of my favourites. It goes something like this:

Once upon a time there was a king with the most amazing palaces, beautiful gardens and parks, servants to cater for his every need and riches beyond his wildest dreams. He did not, however, enjoy good health or happiness. He desired these two qualities more than anything else in life, and sent his servants out far and wide to find someone with the secret that they could share with him. Eventually, after many, many years of combing his kingdom, his servants found an old woman in the mountains who made a very special herbal brew. The King sent for her immediately, but she refused to come, saying that the brew had to be made freshly and the herbs grew only around her small house in the mountains. So one day the King, reluctantly, went to see her. She insisted that he stayed in her house alone with her for a least a week, and again, reluctantly, the King agreed. The old woman gave him simple fresh food and took him for long walks in the beautiful mountains that surrounded her home. They watched the sunrise and sunset and marvelled at the bright starry skies. Each night before bed she dosed him with the special herbal mix, saying it would bring him health and happiness.

The King slept better than he had done in years. At the end of the week, he said happily that the herbal brew had worked wonders and he needed to take a large supply back with him to his palace, for which he would reward her handsomely. The old woman replied, 'There was nothing in the brew that had any special power at all. The secret of happiness and health is and has always been within ourselves.' All she had done was reveal this to him.

Isn't this what we are really looking for? When you are happy and healthy inside, your face and body glow with a youthful inner radiance that no amount of expensive face creams or cosmetic surgery can give you. The Yogis of ancient India realized this well over 5,000 years ago.

What Is Yoga?

The word yoga means 'yoking' or the joining together of body, mind and spirit with the universal spirit. Realizing that for positive health, happiness and peace of mind, both mind and body must work together in complete harmony; the yogis developed this wonderful system of personal development, the science of yoga.

Yoga is comprised of slow, deep, healthy breathing practices to stimulate oxygen to every cell, physical exercises to tone 100 per cent of the body both inside and out, balancing postures to strengthen the body and help us learn the power of concentration and focus, inverted positions to reverse the adverse ageing effects of gravity, stretching movements to keep the joints and spine in perfect condition, deep relaxation to help us release tension and relax, and meditation for calm, deep, inner peace.

The exercises, coupled with a healthy diet, keep the body in radiant health. The body becomes firm and beautiful, the skin glows with health, posture is corrected, stresses and strains vanish, and agility and tremendous flexibility are restored.

In my opinion, yoga is the best elixir of youth. By practising daily you will soon start to reap its magical benefits.

Inside each and every one of us is a force of energy called *prana*, literally translated as 'life-force'. This life-force flows freely through the body in youth, but can dwindle with age if the body isn't cared for correctly, resulting in such things as lack of energy, stiffness in the joints, tension, insomnia, obesity, depression and memory loss, together with poor posture, wrinkled, sagging skin and dull thin hair – i.e., the conditions we refer to as ageing. The modern way of treating this process lies in a special pill, potion, miracle cream or remedy – but these provide only temporary relief, as you are treating the symptoms, not the underlying cause of the problem. The cause is obviously within ourselves.

Yoga proves that with proper exercise it is possible to stimulate the vital force within us. This doesn't come about by applying a miracle cream to your face or by sweating it out in the gym, but by proper breathing, stretching and working your body so that tensions blocking the life-force around every organ, gland, nerve, tendon, cell, blood vessel, joint and bone are released and your body becomes nourished, revitalized and perfectly toned from *within*. This, combined with alleviating stress with deep relaxation and meditation and programming the mind to *think* and *be* 15 years younger, is the real secret to eternal youth.

This wonderful thing called youth cannot be found 'out there', no matter where you look, how many expensive face creams you buy, how far you travel or how much surgery you have. *The secret of youth is within you*.

All you have to do is learn the seven major rejuvenating secrets of yoga and **commit to 15 minutes daily practice seven days a week**, and you will do more for your body, mind, looks and feeling of well-being than you ever thought possible. You will look, feel and be 15 years younger.

The Seven Stay-young Secrets of Yoga

1. The Secret of Energy

The body has a natural energy flow that gives rise to a wonderful feeling of glowing health and well-being. It is, however, easily blocked or interrupted by feelings of tension, worry, anger, guilt, depression, etc. The tensions of the mind can lead to tension in the body, which can weaken the body and can eventually lead to disease.

Yoga gets rid of tension by allowing you to stretch your entire body from top to toe, both inside and out. The deep breathing that accompanies yoga practice increases the oxygen level in the bloodstream. Life-giving oxygen is needed by every cell; the brain in particular has a tremendous need for oxygen.

By stretching out tension, breathing deeply and then performing postures with your head below your heart, oxygen is carefully distributed to all the body's parts, including the brain, and as a result you will feel and look refreshed and revitalized on finishing your yoga workout.

As you continue your yoga practice on a daily basis you will find that your whole body starts to feel better, and you will start to understand that daily stretching to unblock your energy zones, eating fresh, vital foods, learning to relax, and meditating to calm your mind and receive new ideas puts new life into you. The energy of youth is restored and you acquire a new and real zest for life.

An extra benefit comes from visualizing energy flowing through your entire system as you perform your yoga postures. As you concentrate on doing the movements, all negative thoughts will slip from your mind. Negative thoughts are the main energy-drainers, but no matter how tired you are before you start your yoga you will feel calm, focused and energized afterwards. Motion changes emotion.

Whatever you can do or dream you can begin it. Boldness has genius, magic and power in it. Begin it now.

GOETHE

2. The Secret of Perfect Shape

Yoga works 100 per cent of the body, carefully stretching, toning and firming all the muscles in accordance with their natural movements. This gives the body a beautiful shape, corrects posture and rebalances weak areas – correcting ugly, fatty deposits and giving the body the famous streamlined yoga look. Yoga will never give you a hulky-bulky, tight muscular appearance, as this is totally against yoga principles. If you tighten your muscles you are like a puppet whose strings are too taut, inhibiting the natural flexibility of the body and so limiting its movement, leading to unnatural ageing and stiffness.

Firmness of the muscles is essential to prevent the skin sagging and wrinkling and also to keep the internal organs in their correct place. Nothing looks worse than a dropped abdomen, and movements such as the Abdominal Lift are brilliant for keeping this area firm, toned and youthful. The bottom is toned and the back strengthened with movements like the Full Locust. The thighs get an amazing workout with the Camel, Sideways Leg Raise and Heron postures. The arms are perfectly toned with the Chest Expansion, Pose of a Mountain and Cow. The face and neck area become very youthful with the head and neck exercises and the Lion. The hair regains its lustre as the movements stimulate your scalp. Finally, the ageing effects of gravity are carefully reversed by yoga's inverted postures such as the Shoulderstand and Headstand, which do wonders for the way we look and feel.

Grace, beauty, strength, energy and firmness adorn the body through yoga.

YOGA SUTRA III.47

3. The Secret of Concentration and Focus

Once you start yoga, you realize that it is much more than an exercise system. The movements are quite intricate and this necessitates that you give full attention to what you are doing. By concentrating on the movement you are totally involved in the present moment and your mind is given relief from your normal day-to-day activities, so helping it to clear and giving it a rest. This means that after a yoga class your mind is calmer and much more able to deal with everyday problems, and your workload will seem easier. The balances of yoga necessitate total concentration and by focusing on a spot to help us balance physically we calm, clear and balance the mind.

Ayurveda, the holistic medical teaching of ancient India, says 'What you see you become.'

One of yoga's ancient texts puts it this way:

You are what your deep driving desire is. As your desire is so your will, as your will is so is your deed. As your deed is so is your destiny.

BRIHADARANYAKA UPANISHAD IV.4.5

What you see, feel and take in from your environment is a huge amount of stimuli. Your mind cannot possibly take in all this, so it filters out all but a small amount. Your personal selection is very individual and controlled solely by **your** way of interpreting the things around you. For example:

Two people are on holiday abroad together and they go on a tour to see an ancient architectural site. They have to walk about a mile from their coach stop to see this building. It is hot and the road is dusty and dirty; the site, however, is magnificent. On returning to the coach, one person is overjoyed, as the ancient building was bigger, better and more beautiful than her greatest expectations, whereas the other grumbles about the heat, the dust on the road and the dirty, dishevelled appearance of the villagers pestering them to buy souvenirs. She hardly noticed the incredible architecture.

This is just a small example to show how different people can interpret the same experience totally differently. This extraordinary ability of the mind has an incredible effect on our lives, especially with regards to ageing. In his brilliant book, *Grow Younger, Live Longer,* Deepak Chopra tells us of the following experiment.

Harvard psychologist Ellen Langer conducted a fascinating experiment. She took groups of men in their seventies and eighties and encouraged them to think, act and be as if they were 20 years younger. After doing this for only 5 days these men showed a number of physical changes associated with age reversal. Their hearing and vision had improved, they performed better on tests of manual dexterity and joint mobility had improved.

This goes to show that how we think has a huge influence on our body.

Back to the power of focus. If we continually focus on something and keep it in our mind it will grow stronger, whereas if we take our focus away it will gradually wither and disappear. Here is another simple example:

Say you wanted to change your car, and fancied a dark green sports car. You had always wanted a car like this, but only recently felt you could afford it. Every magazine or newspaper you pick up seems to have a dark green sports car in it that catches your eye. As you drive you notice the green sports cars coming in the opposite direction. In car parks you will automatically be drawn to green sports cars.

Now, these cars were there all the time, but you never noticed them because your mind can only take a small selection of the vast amount of stimuli around you. Until you concentrate your mind on something, it does not grow in your consciousness.

We do not see things as they are, we see them as we are.

THE TALMUD

How does this relate to our bodies? Enormously. Every day, focus on excellent health, a beautiful body shape, your body radiant with energy and your life filled with exciting new ideas and projects. See yourself as happy, beautiful, young and vital. As you step into your shower imagine you are stepping into the fountain of youth, which will renew and refresh you daily. Do this every day for a week and you will feel the difference.

Life is the movie you see through your own unique eyes. It makes little difference what is happening out there, it is how you take it that counts.

DENNIS WAITLEY
THE WINNER'S EDGE

4. The Secret of Flexibility

When you meet someone for the very first time, don't you notice their flexibility and posture? Don't you get that feeling of youth and vitality if they stand or sit up straight and move with a relaxed agility? On the other hand, if the person has a stoop and walks stiffly and slowly, don't they immediately look old? The joints and spine normally stiffen with age. Yoga again demonstrates that for life-long flexibility it is necessary to work the joints carefully and in all possible directions of movement. By doing this we stimulate the flow of synovial fluid over the shiny cartilage covering the surfaces of the joints. This acts as 'joint oil' to ensure that the joint moves smoothly, and also gives nourishment to the cartilage. Correct exercise also strengthens the muscles around the joint, giving it support. Yoga will also add to the elasticity of your ligaments and tendons, and can help to remove the calcium deposits that can collect around the joint surface, so helping your joints remain flexible for life.

A major yoga teaching is 'You are as young as your spine is flexible.' This is so true – just look around you and you will find that delightful ageless quality in people with a flexible spine.

The spine has six directions of movement: forwards, backwards, side to side, and twisting in both directions. In our normal waking state, however, over 90 per cent of our time is spent bending forwards. Without correction, this can easily lead to the dreaded stoop. For perfect spinal health and flexibility, the spine needs exercising daily in all six ways. Exercises such as the upward stretch, forwards and backwards bend, or Salute to the Sun, sideways stretch or Half-moon posture and Triangle make a perfect routine that I have recommended to my pupils with back problems for the last 10 years, helping them to achieve amazing success.

For joint flexibility I usually recommend these postures:

o Chest Expansion standing	o Dancer's Posture
o Tree Balance	o Big Toe Balance
o Eagle Balance	o Alternative Leg Pull
o Thigh Stretch	o The Twist
o Backstretch	o The Cow

- The Mountain
- Pose of a Cat
- Pose of a Camel
- Pose of a Dog
  – followed by Deep Relaxation.

If you are really stiff and aching, then it is best to see your doctor in the first instance. With his or her permission, go gently and carefully without strain into each movement. My experience with very many pupils is that yoga's gentle movements can carefully ease the stiffness away and have very beneficial results.

Most people start yoga stiff and uncoordinated, but even after just a few weeks their flexibility improves tremendously, they feel, look and act younger and, as stretching the body releases its tensions, blood flow to the joints is improved, resulting in increased flexibility, healthier joints and the agility of youth.

One of the wonderful things about yoga is that it is never too late, pupils start yoga at all ages and I have many in their late seventies and eighties and all are improving with practice, so **never give up**.

> *A tree that can fill the span of a man's arms grows from a downy tip; a terrace nine storeys high rises from hodfuls of earth; a journey of a thousand miles starts from beneath one's feet.*
>
> LAO TZU, 6TH CENTURY BC

5. The Secret of Perfect Weight

People frequently ask me this question: 'If yoga doesn't burn fat, then how on earth am I going to get slim?'

In yoga, we don't huff and puff with repetitive movements to burn off calories and fat, but instead we work on fine-tuning the entire body, helping it to relaxed, vibrant, positive health.

By working the entire body we stimulate the glands – the Shoulderstand, Fish and Cobra in particular are excellent for stimulating the thyroid gland in the neck, which of course can help energize a sluggish metabolism.

As the body's health improves you will find that your appetite becomes naturally controlled, as your appetite-regulating system works better. You will start to eat less and change to healthier foods. It is difficult to believe, but yoga actually **does** change your taste buds. Pupils frequently tell me that junk food that they thought they couldn't live without now has lost its appeal. As you become healthier, calmer and more relaxed, you will find that you stop 'tension-eating' i.e. grabbing high-calorie snacks at all hours of the day and night.

Yoga's slow stretches give the muscles a beautiful long, lean toned shape, these weigh less than muscles toned by muscle building exercise systems. All this will result in a gradual, natural and healthy return to the best shape possible for your body type for life.

Most people find that gradually over the years their weight normalizes with continued yoga practice, and it does lead people to start considering their diet. They start feeling better and focusing on health, and this leads them into a brand new way of eating. Some pupils, however, have been steeped in bad eating habits for so long that they need a lot of guidance before change can be effected. Because of this I offer the following advice.

1. DON'T EAT STANDING UP

Obey this rule for one week and see the difference! So many people constantly nibble, eating on the go, eating between meals, eating the kids' leftovers, 'tasting' as they cook the dinner, etc. This means that they are never really hungry and are always amazed when their skinny friends say, 'I'm starving' and sit and eat a good meal. When you stop picking and nibbling, your appetite will become fine-tuned and you will enjoy your food so much more. Everything tastes great when you are really hungry. You will also know exactly what you eat and stop kidding yourself that you eat like a bird.

2. NEVER EAT BETWEEN MEALS

Again, a continuation of the rule above, this stops the constant nibbling and snacking. When you sit down and eat three meals a day calmly and slowly with nothing in between you will find it makes a huge difference to your weight and the way you feel. You will feel so much more in control!

3. NEVER MORE THAN HALF-FILL YOUR STOMACH WITH FOOD; LEAVE A QUARTER FOR FLUID AND A QUARTER FOR DIGESTION

This is brilliant advice from yoga's ancient texts (Hatha Yoga Pradipika 4.58). Now let's recap – if you don't eat standing up and don't eat between meals, you eat slowly and calmly, and never more than half-fill your stomach with food, you will normally find any excess weight slipping away naturally.

What to Eat

In yoga we eat for total positive health and for stimulating the *prana* or life-force within us. This is pure, natural food. Prepare your meals from the following selections: Feast on beautiful fresh fruit and natural healthy juices, fresh vegetables and salads, enjoy natural whole grains, nuts and seeds, a little milk, butter, cheese, natural organic live yoghurt, eggs, moderate amounts of fish and chicken and a small amount of red meat. Olive oil and walnut oil are excellent for inclusion in salad dressings with either lemon juice or vinegar, and be sure to add fresh herbs and spices to flavour your food. Try to drink at least 2 litres of water per day, and enjoy herbal tea and natural fruit juices. Try to restrict coffee and tea to a maximum of five cups per day, and have decaffeinated if possible. Restrict alcohol to just 1 glass of wine a day if desired.

Avoid all diet products (they may contain additives; it is best to just eat fresh natural healthy food), biscuits, cakes, sweets, chocolates, bagels, buns, pasta (apart from wholegrain), pizza, jelly, blancmange and ice cream. Puddings, packaged cereals (apart from organic wholegrain ones), jams, sandwich spreads and fillers, fizzy drinks and heat-and-serve meals won't do you any favours. Keep the accent on fresh, fresh, fresh foods – nothing tinned, frozen or preserved. (I have never seen a slim person asking for a diet drink or using sweeteners, but I find my larger friends use diet products constantly.)

Think back to our Stone Age ancestors. They could only eat food that they could grow, catch or trap – no preservatives or additives were around, just a pure, natural, healthy diet. This is obviously the diet nature intended for us.

Finally, my advice to you is make your own menu plans from the foods advised – and *enjoy* your food. If you find your weight not slipping away as you wish, simply cut down on your portions. I know it may seem hard, but once you realize that if you are heavier than your ideal weight for your height and build, quite simply *eating less* will do the trick.

> *Man lives on one-quarter of what he eats. On the other three quarters his doctor lives.*
> CHISELLED 5,000 YEARS AGO ON A PYRAMID IN EGYPT

You don't have to gain weight as you get older. *Please* don't believe the excuses. Eating less is healthier; you feel better and have more energy. I could write an entire book on excuses people have given me as to why they are fat. Here are just a few examples:

o   It's a choice between face or figure after 40.
o   It's hereditary.
o   It's my bone structure.
o   It's my hormones.
o   If I lose weight I'll look too thin in the face.
o   It's my glands.
o   My friends tell me I look great at a size 18 (at 5'4"?).
o   It's my HRT.
o   It's because I'm on the pill.
o   I retain water, it's not really fat.
o   I hardly eat anything – I get fat if I just *look* at a piece of cake.
o   It's because I had that operation.
o   Ever since I had my baby, my body shape has changed (no but your eating habits did!).

Fools need to know that half exceeds the whole, how blest the sparing meal and temperate bowl.

HESIOD, 700BC

While there may be a small amount of truth in some of the above claims, I do find that for the majority of people, sticking to the above rules will do the trick. It is possible to keep your body in perfect shape regardless of age, and the food guide above will add to your health and vitality, and make you look and feel much younger. Doctors now tell us that the overload of toxins, chemicals, E numbers and preservatives in our food can contribute to wrinkled skin, grey hair and stiff joints. In his wonderful book *Perfect Health*, Deepak Chopra says, 'Your adipose tissue (fat cells) fill up with fat and empty out constantly so all of it is exchanged every three weeks. You acquire a new stomach lining every five days (the innermost layer of stomach cells also is exchanged in a matter of minutes as you digest your food). Your skin is new every five weeks. Your skeleton, seemingly so solid and rigid, is entirely new every 3 months.'

So, as your body is being renewed all the time, why not change from being overweight and accepting illness, degeneration and decay, and help your body to vital positive health, youth, great hair, beautiful skin, good strong bones and a fabulous body?

Change to the above plan and sit back and wait for the compliments to roll in.

A final tip: Search through the magazines and find a body you really would love to have. Cut it out and paste it in your notebook or diary or on a piece of thin white cardboard – the card they put inside packets of tights is just perfect. Find a photo of you smiling, and replace the model's head with your own. Don't you look fantastic?! Keep this picture with you and look at it at least three times a day, before breakfast, lunch and dinner. This will imprint your new image deep into your subconscious mind, making it your real new image of you (more about this in the Meditation chapter); it will also stop you overeating.
Good luck and good health!

Menu Plan
On the opposite page I have planned your first week's diet for you. You may start on any day and interchange the menus to suit your own personal requirements. By following the plan shown you should easily lose at least 2–3 lb a week.

Caution: **I advise you to consult your doctor or nutritionist before starting on this or any other eating plan, to make sure that it is suitable for your personal dietary requirements.**

Let your food be your medicine; let your medicine be your food.   HIPPOCRATES

Remember, the body you will wear tomorrow will be made of the food you eat today!

Sunday	Monday	Tuesday	Wednesday	Thursday	Friday	Saturday
Breakfast						
1 carton natural organic yoghurt, 1 carton fresh raspberries	½ grapefruit, 1 slice whole-grain toast & a little butter	1 glass fresh orange juice, 1 carton natural organic yoghurt	1 slice whole-grain toast & a little butter, 1 large slice melon	1 poached egg & 1 slice wholegrain toast & butter	1 carton fresh straw-berries, 1 carton of natural organic yoghurt	1 banana, 1 small mango
Lunch						
2 slices roast lamb, gravy, mint sauce, carrots, runner beans; 1 apple	3oz tuna fish, large salad of lettuce, tomato, cucumber, black olives, 1 tbsp oil & vinegar dressing; 1 pear	Prawn & salad sandwich made with 2 slices whole-grain bread, 3 oz prawns, 1 dessert spoon mayonnaise plus a little mixed salad	Salad made from ½ avocado, fresh spinach, 3 rashers bacon, 1 tbsp oil & vinegar dressing	1 glass tomato juice, 6oz cottage cheese, salad made with lettuce, tomato, cucumber, grated carrot plus 1 tbsp mayonnaise or oil & vine-gar dressing	1 glass fresh mixed fruit juice, ½ avocado, 2 tomatoes, 3oz mozzarella with salad & 1 tbsp dressing	Caesar salad made with 2 oz parme-san cheese, cos lettuce, ½ slice wholegrain bread made into croutons with 1 tbsp dressing
Dinner						
Fresh asparagus, grilled plaice, mixed salad, 1 tbsp oil & vinegar dressing	1 large breast grilled chicken, broccoli in a little cheese sauce, with 2 grilled tomatoes	3–4oz grilled salmon, fresh spinach, large mixed salad & 1 tbsp dressing; 1 fresh fig	1 bowl fresh mussels in white wine sauce with garlic, large mixed salad and 1 tbsp dressing	Roast chicken, swede, French beans, gravy & 1 tsp cranberry sauce; 1 fresh peach	Melon; grilled lean pork chop and apple sauce, courgettes, 4 grilled mushrooms with garlic	4 King Prawns in a little garlic butter, 4 oz beef steak, mixed salad, 1 tbsp dress-ing

Rules

8 glasses water per day or more if desired. Tea and coffee limit to 5 cups per day and try to restrict to decaffeinated, with milk from allowance. Unlimited herbal tea. 1 glass wine per day if desired. Half-pint semi-skimmed milk or soya milk. Salad dressing – make fresh from olive oil or walnut oil, lemon juice or vinegar, a little garlic and/or fresh herbs.

6. The Secret of Deep Relaxation and Meditation

One of the main reasons for our survival as a species is our incredible 'fight or flight' response to sudden danger.

Putting it simply, in ancient times if a wild animal suddenly started to chase our Stone Age ancestor (let's call him Fred), his body would react in the following way to the danger: His mind would fill with fear, adrenaline would be secreted, his blood sugar would go up, the blood supply to his muscles would increase, his muscles would tense, the blood-clotting mechanism would kick in, enabling his body to heal faster in case of injury, his breathing would become rapid and shallow, his brain would become hyper-alert, his digestion would be suppressed (his body knowing this is no time for a sandwich), his sexual desire would be suppressed (not the time to make love), his blood vessels would tighten to enable blood to flow through them faster and his blood pressure would increase, his immune system would be suppressed (this is no time to worry about a virus), more oxygen would be consumed and more carbon dioxide would be expelled. Fred is then programmed to look and be alert for more danger. In normal times, a huge percentage of cellular energy goes into building new cells, but during the fight-or-flight response energy is poured into the muscles, with the result that eventually tissue breakdown can occur.

This reaction is brilliant if Fred has to run or fight. Fred – and all of us – need this reaction to sudden danger as it gives us the incredible extra power and energy we need to react in an emergency, e.g. saving someone from drowning.

Nowadays, thank goodness, sudden danger is relatively rare, but the body's reaction to a stressful event continues. And whereas we all have to be grateful to it for our survival as a species, now this reaction can be the cause of major health problems due to the modern-day overload of mental stress.

Doctors now realize that very many diseases are caused by stress. The problem is the body still reacts in this same way to the normal stresses of everyday life. For example, if you are late for a big meeting, you burn the dinner at an important dinner party, the dry cleaners ruin your best suit, you car won't start or your son fails his final exams (the list is endless and is quite simply called 'life'), you react with the physical changes listed above. This stress reaction, if not balanced by periods of relaxation, can now start to weaken the body and may give rise to such things as menstrual problems, high blood pressure, chronic fatigue, gastric ulcer, lower disease resistance, frequent headaches, cancer and heart attack, and makes us look and feel much older than our years.

Unless we make a conscious effort to control our stress levels, it is easy to let the stress response take hold. This is why yoga does us so much good and helps us live comfortably and easily in today's high-pressure world.

Yoga's wonderful stretches release the chronic tension that is held within your body. By deep breathing in every posture you stimulate life-giving oxygen to every cell. The act of slow, deep breathing also calms your mind and aids deep relaxation. By concentrating on the balancing movements you take your mind off its troubles, allowing it to calm and feel peaceful. Relaxing at the end of yoga practice allows the stresses of the day to gently float away, and frequent practice of meditation brings inner peace. As a result, the mind becomes clearer and calmer, muscular tension decreases, the secretion of adrenaline is lowered and breathing slows down. The heart rate slows, blood pressure normalizes and the blood-clotting mechanism is gently reduced, sweating gently ceases and the body becomes cooled and calmed, and digestion and the immune system are relaxed and restored to normal.

This relaxation has a most wonderful effect on your looks, as the tension around the arteries relaxes; the blood flow to the skin is restored, giving the skin back its beautiful healthy glow. Blood flow to the hair follicles is increased due to tension release, so improving the condition of the hair, frown lines are smoothed and you both look and feel wonderful, radiant and much younger.

Our greatest experiences are our quietest moments.

NIETZSCHE (1844–1900)

7. The Secret of Radiant Health

These days everything comes with a manual – 60 pages just on the use of a mobile phone, 100 pages with a recipe book for your food mixer, a large manual for your washing machine and a huge manual for your car. The most complex and brilliant system in your house, however, is your own body – and sadly we are born without a manual!

Wouldn't it be wonderful if we did have a manual to instruct us on how to keep the body in perfect condition? We would then know how to care for all of the body's complex systems and keep them in perfect health. We would know how to oil our joints to keep them flexible, how to move our spine in all six directions to prevent it becoming stiff and aching, we would practise weight-bearing movements to strengthen our bones and we would learn beautiful stretches to keep our muscles in perfect shape.

EATING CORRECTLY

We would learn to eat correctly and never too much so that we never overloaded our stomach, heart, lungs, joints and internal organs. We would then eat foods with health and vitality in mind rather than filling our bodies with junk and toxins that our bodies have no use for and find it difficult to remove.

FRESH AIR

We would learn the necessity of beautiful fresh air and correct breathing to make full use of our lungs and absorb more oxygen into our system. We would learn movements to get rid of tightness in our chest and calm our mind with slow, calm, relaxing breathing.

GOOD DIGESTION

We would learn how to keep our digestive system in good shape, never overloading it, and we would appreciate the importance of movements to massage the digestive system such as the abdominal lift and contractions and the spinal twists and upwards stretch and forwards and backwards bend. We would learn the effect of stress on the digestive system and realize the importance of relaxation to release the adverse effects of tension on our digestive organs.

CIRCULATORY HEALTH

We would learn to care for our heart and blood vessels. Under stress, the body tries to make an enormous amount of energy available to enable us to flee or fight. This accelerates the heart rate and also squeezes the arteries and veins to try to raise the rate at which the blood flows through, and as a result the blood pressure is raised. The clotting mechanism of the blood is also raised, as the body sensibly thinks that if one has to flee or fight, an injury could be a likely outcome.

The net result of this is that the heart pumps thickened blood faster through narrow tubes. Because of this pressure, when the body is under long-term stress the arterial walls frequently become damaged. As the body tries its hardest to repair itself no matter how badly we treat it, it sends blood platelets and fatty acids to seal the damage; this, however, results in narrowing the arteries further. Continued stress increases the clotting mechanism, and if a clot breaks loose it can easily block a narrowed blood vessel. This, of course, can be fatal. So if we learn to stretch away our tensions daily, eat a healthy diet and relax and allow our arteries and blood-clotting mechanism to calm down, the fight-or-flight reaction subsides, the blood-clotting mechanism is lowered, the arteries relax and blood pressure returns to normal. This would result in excellent care of our heart and circulatory system.

THE GLANDULAR SYSTEM

Our ductless glands control the amazing chemistry of our bodies, carefully regulating and controlling the mind–body relationship. If our body manual taught us that the detrimental effect of stress can upset our entire glandular system, we would understand how the pituitary – the master gland of the body – controls the secretions of all the other glands. In yoga we help balance the pituitary with the Headstand. The thyroid gland controls our metabolism, and the parathyroids control the calcium and phosphate level in the blood. The most important exercises for these glands are the Shoulderstand and the Fish. The sex hormones, if imbalanced, can lead to menstrual problems and infertility in women, and fertility problems in men. The Cobra, Bow, Locust and deep relaxation help these areas tremendously.

The adrenal glands, together with the sex hormones and corticosteroids, produce adrenalin to arouse the body to flee or fight. These glands are kept in excellent condition by movements such as the Cobra, Crescent Moon and Camel. Deep relaxation and meditation also relieve the stress that arouses this reaction. The pancreas is essential for the production of insulin to regulate the blood sugar of the body. The Pose of a Peacock and the Spinal Twist help balance this organ – and again, a healthy natural diet stops to body from overloading with excess sugar.

THE BRAIN AND SPINAL CORD

Finally, with the help of our body manual we could learn how to control our nervous system and realize the incredible importance of our brain and spinal cord.

As you will see from Figure 1, 'The chiropractor's view of the spine', the 31 pairs of spinal nerves exit from the spinal cord supplying every part of the body. Tension around these nerves weakens the area they supply, with the resulting problems indicated. By performing your yoga stretches daily and learning to relax, you will relieve the tension from the roots of these nerves and encourage their correct functioning. Daily relaxation is of prime importance – during relaxation the mind calms and pressure on the spinal nerves is released.

The calming effect of yoga movements also balances the involuntary symptoms of the fight-or-flight reaction, calming and cooling the body and thus reducing the adverse effects of chronic stress.

Figure 1
The chiropractor's
view of the spine

Cervical
Spine

Thoracic
Spine

Lumbar
Spine

Sacral

VERTEBRAE	AREAS AND PARTS OF BODY	POSSIBLE SYMPTOMS
C1	Blood supply to the head, brain, scalp, pituitary gland, bones of the face, inner and middle ear, sympathetic nervous system	Headaches, insomnia, nervousness, high blood pressure, head colds, migraine headaches, nervous breakdowns, chronic tiredness, amnesia, dizziness
C2	Eyes, optic nerves, auditory nerves, mastoid bones, sinuses, forehead, tongue	Allergies, sinus trouble, pain around the eyes, fainting spells, earache, certain cases of blindness, crossed eyes, deafness
C3	Cheeks, face bones, outer ear, teeth, trifacial nerve	Neuralgia, acne or pimples, neuritis, eczema
C4	Lips, nose, eustachian tube, mouth	Runny nose, hay fever, hearing loss, adenoids
C5	Vocal cords, glands, neck, pharynx	Hoarseness, laryngitis, throat conditions such as sore throat or quinsy
C6	Neck muscles, tonsils, shoulders	Pain in upper arm, stiff neck, tonsillitis, croup, chronic cough
C7	Bursae in the shoulders, thyroid gland, elbows	Colds, bursitis, thyroid conditions
T1	Arms from the elbows down, including hands, wrists and fingers, oesophagus and trachea	Asthma, cough, shortness of breath, difficult breathing, pain in lower arm and hands
T2	Heart, including its valves and covering, coronary arteries	Functional heart conditions and certain chest conditions
T3	Lungs, pleura, bronchial tubes, chest, breast	Bronchitis, pneumonia, pleurisy, congestion, influenza
T4	Common duct, gall bladder	Gall bladder conditions, shingles, jaundice
T5	Solar plexus, liver, circulation (general)	Fevers, liver conditions, blood pressure problems, poor circulation, arthritis
T6	Stomach	Stomach troubles, including nervous stomach, heartburn, indigestion, dyspepsia
T7	Duodenum, pancreas	Gastritis, ulcers
T8	Spleen	Lowered resistance
T9	Adrenal and supra-renal glands	Allergies, hives
T10	Kidneys	Kidney troubles, hardening of the arteries, chronic tiredness, pyelitis, nephritis
T11	Kidneys, ureters	Skin conditions such as acne, pimples, boils, eczema
T12	Small intestines, lymph circulation	Rheumatism, gas pains, certain types of sterility
L1	Large intestines, inguinal rings	Constipation, dysentery, colitis, diarrhea, some ruptures or hernias
L2	Appendix, abdomen, upper leg	Difficult breathing, cramps, minor varicose veins
L3	Sex organs, uterus, bladder, knees	Bladder troubles, menstrual problems such as painful or irregular periods, bedwetting, miscarriages, impotence, change of life symptoms, many knee pains
L4	Prostate gland, muscles of the lower back, sciatic nerve	Lumbago, sciatica, difficult, painful or too frequent urination, backaches
L5	Lower legs, feet, ankles	Poor circulation in the legs, swollen ankles, weak ankles and arches, cold feet, leg cramps, weakness in the legs
Sacrum	Hip bones, buttocks	Sacro-iliac conditions, spinal curvatures
Coccyx	Rectum, anus	Haemorrhoids (piles), pruritis (itching), pain at end of spine on sitting

Your Personal Manual for Health

In the pages that follow you will be treated to your personal health manual and learn that by looking after your body, exercising it, eating fresh natural foods, breathing correctly, learning to relax and cope with stress, concentrating your mind on what you want rather than what you *don't* want, and keeping your joints and spine flexible and tension-free, you will look and feel 15 years younger in 15 minutes a day.

The manual for this is the secret of health and vitality for ever, and was discovered over 5,000 years ago, and is and always will be YOGA.

The Rejuvenating Benefits of Yoga

1. Yoga improves the flexibility and strength of the spine, so helping to prevent back problems.
2. Yoga oils the joints, keeping them flexible and so helping to prevent aches, pain and stiffness.
3. Yoga releases tension in the neck and shoulders, so helping to prevent headaches and the proverbial 'pain in the neck'.
4. Yoga corrects poor posture, so helping to prevent the dreaded stoop.
5. Yoga means daily exercises to keep the body in perfect shape and condition instead of having to worry about uneven fatty deposits and middle-age spread.
6. Yoga means eating for health and vitality and enjoying a slim beautiful shape, instead of consuming an overload of junk and being constantly on a diet.
7. Yoga means enjoying the present moment instead of wasting time worrying about yesterday or feeling anxious about tomorrow.
8. Yoga means slow, deep breathing to energize every cell in the body and calm and relax the mind, freeing you from low energy levels, nervousness and breathing difficulties.
9. Yoga releases tension in the lower abdomen, so helping to prevent constipation and period pains.
10. Yoga strengthens the bones, so helping to prevent osteoporosis.
11. Yoga means taking time out to relax, calm the mind and refocus instead of falling prey to chronic stress-related diseases.
12. To sum up, yoga is being in control, creating the mind, body and life you desire, looking younger, feeling better and enjoying life more than ever before.

Before We Begin

I do hope that you are now really raring to go and can't wait to get started. Just before we begin, however, a few guidelines for your yoga practice:

1. Work in a warm, airy room in bare feet and wear loose comfortable clothing. A leotard and tights are in my opinion the best for women, but jogging bottoms and t-shirts are also fine, and are the best option for men.
2. Wait until at least two hours after a main meal before you practise yoga.
3. Make sure that you won't be disturbed. You deserve time just for yourself to concentrate your body and clear your mind.
4. You will need a mat or blanket to sit on. Yoga is very much a 'no-equipment' exercise system, so you don't even need to buy a special mat for your yoga. A blanket has always been the traditional suggestion for yoga practice, but if you haven't got one that you feel is suitable, a car rug or thick bath towel will do fine. There are now many yoga mats on the market that some people find useful, but I am a bit of a traditionalist and still prefer my blanket.
5. Yoga is great for all age groups – my pupils range from 4 to 84 – however, it is for healthy people, so if you do have any health concerns whatsoever, just ask your doctor's advice before you begin. If your doctor is unclear about the type of movements you will be doing, take this book along to show him, but do emphasize that you will not be straining and will only be moving into the positions at your own pace, going into your maximum position in each movement. **You must have your doctor's consent before you start to practise.** Yoga is very beneficial for your health and frequently many health problems can be greatly helped by yoga practice. You must however never substitute yoga for your doctor's treatment.
6. PREGNANCY: Yoga can be most beneficial during both pregnancy and labour. However, if you are new to yoga, I recommend waiting until after your 3-month check-up at about 14–15 weeks before commencing yoga practice. If you have been practising yoga on a regular basis prior to conception and have no history of miscarriage then there should be no reason why you should not continue. **You must always make sure that your doctor gives you permission to practise yoga during pregnancy.**

    I do prefer that you go to a class qualified to guide you through the various stages of pregnancy as the movements need to be adjusted to cope with the baby's increasing size. In general, avoid all the movements which put strain on the abdomen (these are indicated throughout the book) and always move carefully and slowly without strain. Learn to relax and enjoy your pregnancy.

    Following the birth, it is advisable to wait until your post-natal check-up before resuming yoga practice. If your doctor is happy that all is well and gives you his blessing to recommence practice then do tell your teacher of the nature of your delivery. Start very gently and carefully. You will quickly regain your shape and feeling of well-being.

The golden rule of yoga: Never, ever strain. I know this is different from other methods of exercise that you might have tried, but in yoga we focus on the positive health of the pupil and the enhancement of the energy flow or life-force within us. Straining in yoga is never an option.

Your body today is the result of how it has been taken care of, how you have exercised, coped with your share of troubles, the diet you have eaten, how you have slept and relaxed and your individual focus and attitude to life.

It is extremely hard to suddenly come face-to-face with your body in certain movements and realize how stiff and out of shape and uncoordinated you have become. Please cheer up – it really is a good thing to gradually discover our imbalances and frailties. All you need is your daily yoga to help correct them.

Now, to go back to straining – if you strain or jerk in a movement you are liable to tear or hurt yourself, so putting a total halt on further practice for a while.

Move into each posture slowly and carefully without strain, and relax in your own maximum position. This is the secret of success. Every time you practise, no matter how bad you were to start with, you will find that you are a tiny bit more flexible, and after just a few weeks you will really see the difference in your flexibility, shape and feeling of well-being. When a system has been tried and tested for over 5,000 years, as yoga has, and is still increasing in popularity, **we know it works!**

> *The key to developing a beautiful physical appearance is to start from the inside out by clearing away physical and emotional toxins.*
>
> ANNE LOUISE GITTLEMAN

How to Use
This Book

Decide now to devote a minimum of 15 minutes a day to your yoga practice. Decide on the time of day convenient for practice, and commit to it.

Start with Stage 1 of '15-Minute Miracles' and do it every day, if possible before breakfast. As soon as it becomes really easy, then move on to Stage 2, which is a little stronger, and finally to Stage 3. Stages 4, 5 and 6 are ideal to do in the afternoon or in the evening before bed. Try them in the same way as the earlier Stages, moving at your own pace.
Find a time that suits your schedule. If, like me, you are a morning type, then just do either the a.m. or p.m. workouts in the morning, or both if you have time.

Continue in this way until you are able to do all six Stages with ease. This will give you a fantastic grounding in yoga and will tone and firm all the major muscles in your body and leave you feeling relaxed, calm and revitalized, and much, much younger.

Once you have mastered these Stages, replace them on alternate days with your own choice of the first four sequences in Part Two – concentrating on your face, arms/neck/shoulders, stomach, and bottom/hips/thighs – which will help perfect your body in record time:

o   Your 15-minute facial will sculpt and tone your facial muscles, neck and jaw, while releasing neck tension. The eye exercises will help your vision and eye muscle tone. Once learned, all these movements can be done at odd moments during the day.
o   The arms, neck and shoulders movements are excellent for toning and firming the arms and shoulders, and also firm the bust and help to relieve neck and shoulder tension.
o   The flat stomach plan is an amazing system for giving you a firm, flat tummy. It consists of movements already included in the first six Stages, grouped for easy reference should you wish to have that flat tummy in record time.
o   The bottom, hips and thighs plan is composed of two 15-minute sequences of movements that you will already have practised. If this area is a challenging one for you, these movements will sculpt your hips, bottom and thighs and really benefit your shape and reduce cellulite. Again, use it as well as or alternating with the 15-Minute Miracles.

When you feel ready, move on to 'Your Ageless Body'. These movements are amazing. I show you how, with continued practice 15 minutes a day, you can reap yoga's wonderful benefits: an ageless body and mind. Personally I would hate to grow old without yoga. I am delighted to show you these movements and to show you how you can be in great shape and feeling and looking fantastic at any age.

In the Age-defying Anti-gravity Movements section, you will learn that these postures are quite simply the best face-lift in the world, doing wonders for your skin, hair, brain, energy level and feeling of well-being.

Until you are familiar with the movements in all six Stages and beyond, you may like to tape-record yourself reading the instructions for each posture, or do them with a friend, taking it in turns to read out the instructions to each other. Then, once you are familiar with the names and sequence of movements for each posture, you can make up a schedule or chart for yourself for each daily 15-minute sequence, using just the names of the postures as your guide.

The final three chapters of this book focus on techniques to help you get the most out of life alongside your daily yoga practice:

o   The Meditation chapter will help you to learn the amazing benefits of simple meditation exercises.
o   In the Visualization chapter, we focus on your life and goals – to help you to reach them.
o   Finally, the last chapter offers you my 30 Top Tips to help you look and stay young for ever.

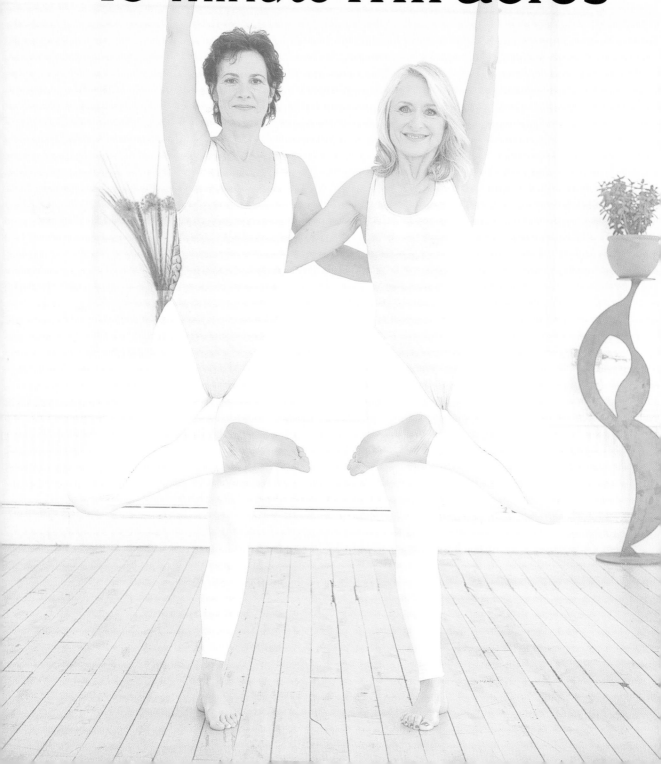

Part One

15-minute **miracles**

15-Minute Miracles
Stage 1

This sequence will start to correct your posture, tone and firm your upper arms and neck, help your spine to incredible flexibility, slim your midriff, waistline, thighs and upper arms, aid joint flexibility and help you to develop the powers of focus and concentration.

- Breathing Demonstration
- Free the Spirit Standing
- Posture Clasp Standing
- Sideways Stretch
- Upwards Stretch Forwards and Backwards Bend
- Rishis Posture
- Body Roll
- Awkward Posture
- Toe Balance
- Tree Balance

True beauty must come, must be grown, from within ...
RALPH W TRINE (1866–1958)

1　Breathing Demonstration

Good deep breathing while performing the yoga movements is very important, as it stimulates your entire body with life-giving oxygen.

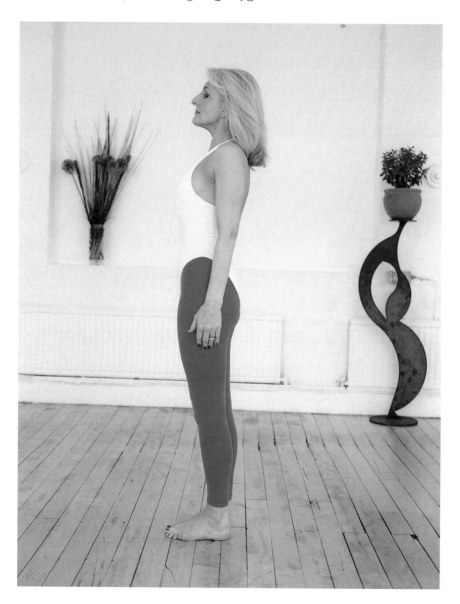

- In general, gently push your abdominal muscles out and inhale slowly through your nose as you start to stretch into the posture.
- As you move into the movement, slowly and calmly exhale through your nose.
- Whilst relaxing in the movement, just breathe normally and peacefully through your nose.

2 Free the Spirit Standing

This movement gives you instant stress relief, literally making you feel free from all limitations. It is great if you have been hunched over your desk for any length of time. It also helps correct your posture, release shoulder tension and firm your throat and jaw line.

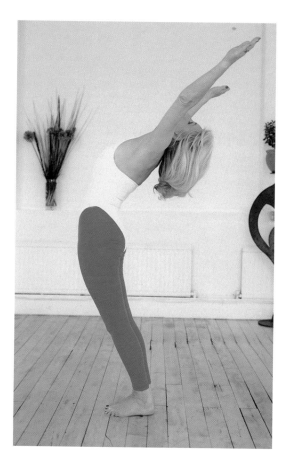 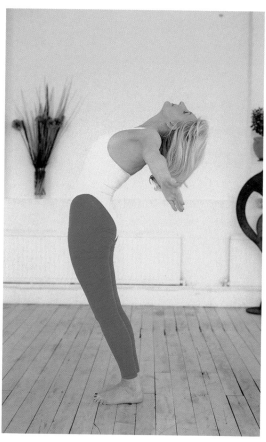

- Stand straight, shoulders back, feet together and correct your posture. Hold your hands as if in prayer. Inhale and lift your arms up straight in front of you until they are pointing towards the ceiling. Drop your head gently backwards and, keeping it back, open your arms wide.

- Making the widest circle possible, lower your arms down to your sides while exhaling very slowly. Repeat three times.

3   Posture Clasp Standing

How I wish this was taught in school! This clever movement restores balance to your shoulders, corrects posture, firms the muscles of the upper arms, tones the pectoral muscles that support the bust and releases shoulder tension.

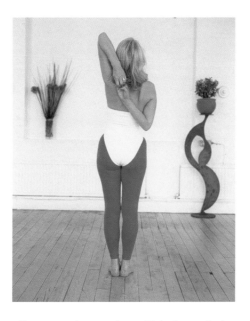

- Stand straight with your feet together and shoulders back. Inhale and lift your left arm in the air, then drop it back. Take your right hand down and stretch it behind your back. Aim to join your hands together with the fingers clasped as shown.

- Exhale and, breathing normally, hold your maximum movement in this position for a count of 5.
- Unclasp your hands and repeat to the other side. Repeat the entire sequence twice.

Help and Advice

This movement can be a nasty shock: sometimes it appears impossible on both sides, sometimes one side is relatively easy and the other side is impossible, even though you are using the same pair of arms! Cheer up! Hardly anyone can manage this movement on both sides to begin with. Over the years our shoulders become imbalanced due to many things, including carrying a heavy briefcase, slinging a shoulder bag over one shoulder, using the right arm more than the left, constant use of the telephone, slumping over your desk or computer, etc., etc. However, one of the most important things to correct is your posture, as over the years this can gradually get worse and worse resulting in the dreaded stoop and dowager's hump. By doing this simple movement daily twice on each side without strain, you will gradually correct your posture. You will also become more posture-conscious and find you start noticing how other people walk and carry themselves. Very gradually, even if your hands were miles apart in the beginning, you will find that they will soon join up.

4   Sideways Stretch

This movement is great for slimming and toning the midriff and waistline, giving the spine tremendous flexibility and releasing tension in the lower back.

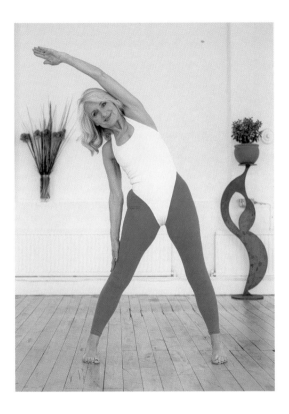

- Stand straight with your feet facing forwards and about 3 feet apart. Breathe in and lift your left hand in the air.
- Exhale and, keeping your body in line, slide your right hand down your right leg as far as possible. Keep your left arm straight, with the inner part of your left arm close to your left ear.
- Hold your maximum stretch for a count of 5. Inhale and, slowly and smoothly, return to an upright position. Exhale, slowly lower your arm and relax. Repeat the movement on the other side, then repeat the entire sequence twice.

Help and Advice
There is a huge temptation to bend forwards in this movement to get your hand further down the leg. Please don't. Keep your body straight and keep looking forwards. This slow, careful movement is excellent for toning and slimming your midriff and waistline.

'I have suffered for many years with neck, shoulder and back problems and found no improvement or relief after consulting various medical specialists. However, within a month of starting yoga I noticed a great improvement with pain relief and posture. Now, after a year of yoga, I have become very flexible and found my waistline, which I didn't know existed.'

ANN, 42

5 Upward Stretch Forwards and Backwards Bend

This brilliant revitalizing morning stretch releases tension from the entire body, corrects posture and gives amazing flexibility to the spine. It slims and tones the abdomen, midriff, waistline and throat, and firms and tones the backs of the thighs and calves. By encouraging blood flow to the head and neck area, it boosts the condition of the skin, hair and brain cells.

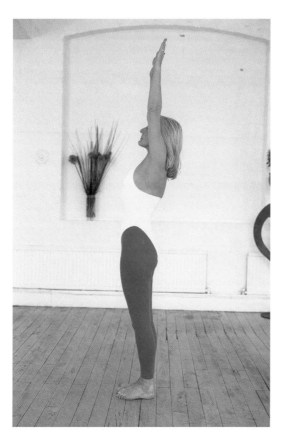

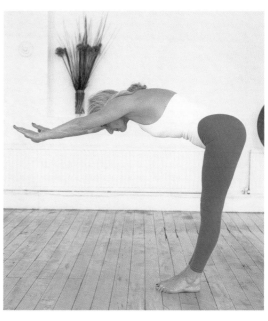

• Exhale slowly as you move forwards, keeping your back flat and your legs straight. Don't strain. Relax in your maximum position and hold the movement for a count of 5, breathing normally.

• Stand straight with your feet facing forwards and about 12 inches apart. Correct your posture. Inhale and lift your arms straight up above your head.

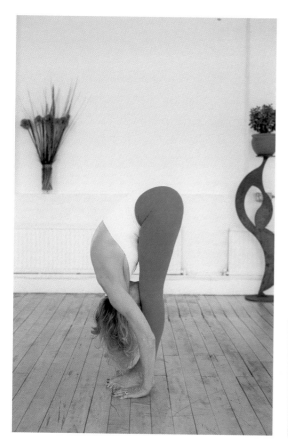

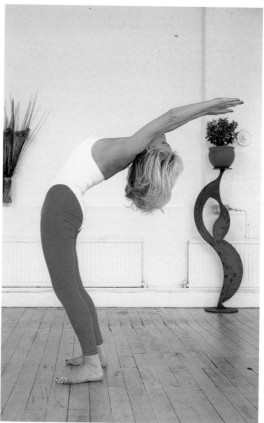

- Your eventual aim is to have your hands flat on the floor and your chin on your shins. Inhale and lift your head first and then, slowly, keeping your back flat and legs straight, return to an upright position.

- Stretch your arms up above your head and, keeping your eyes on your thumbs, slowly, without strain, relax backwards, exhaling in your maximum position. Hold for a count of 5. Your eventual aim is a beautiful backwards arch as shown. Inhale as you slowly return to an upright position. Exhale, lower your arms, and relax. Repeat twice.

Help and Advice

It's not until we start to work the spine that we realize just how stiff we have become. I know, I have been there!

The body operates on a 'use it or lose it' system, but even if you are totally stiff to start with, with daily practice even the stiffest back can regain its youthful flexibility. Remember not to strain, relax in your own maximum position even if you can move very little in the beginning, and you will be delighted at how quickly your flexibility will improve and how much better you will feel.

Moving backwards for the first time can present a huge challenge, but keep your eyes on your thumbs, relax and, even if you only move an inch back in the beginning stages, with practice this will improve very quickly – I promise.

6   Rishis Posture

This movement is brilliant for releasing deep-seated tension and rebalancing the lower back. I really recommend it for people with 'lop-sided' jobs, e.g. dentists or people who play imbalanced sports such as tennis or golf. Gardeners can find it really helpful to release the tension resulting from being in awkward positions for a considerable length of time. This posture will tone and firm your midriff and waistline, bottom and thighs, and keep your back in great condition, enhancing its flexibility. It relieves tension from the chest and firms your jaw and throat.

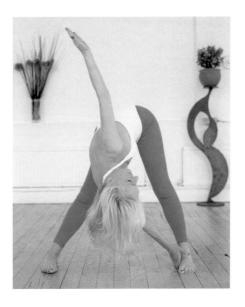

- Stand straight with perfect posture, your feet 3 feet apart with your toes facing forwards, not outwards. Lift your arms straight up in the air as you inhale. As you exhale, with your back flat and your legs straight, move forwards to your own maximum position without strain. Slide your right hand to your left leg, grabbing it wherever comfortable – but don't bend your knees. Eventually your aim is to place your right hand under your left foot. Lift your left arm in the air; now, slowly and carefully, turn your body so that you are looking at your left hand. Hold this position for a count of 5, breathing normally, then slowly lower your arm and relax forwards.

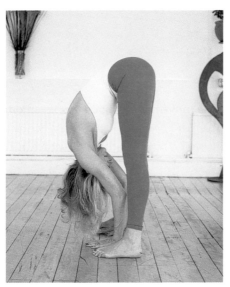

- Now repeat to the other side, sliding your left hand to your maximum position on your right leg and lifting your right arm in the air. Hold for a count of 5, then slowly lower your arm and let your body relax in its maximum forwards bend. Hold this position for a count of 5, breathing normally. Grab your legs and – gently, keeping your back straight – draw your body inwards towards your legs and then relax, aiming to place your hands on the floor.

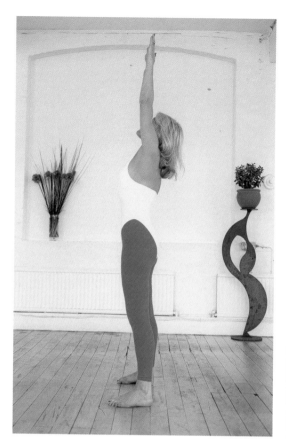

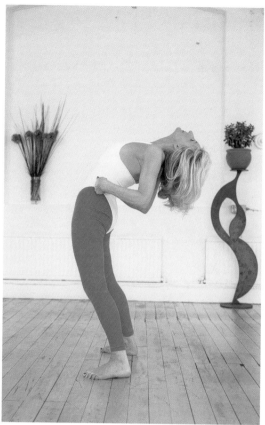

- Inhale deeply and lift your head, then slowly return to an upright position and stretch your arms up above your head.

- Now place your hands at your waistline with your thumbs in front and fingers behind. Inhale deeply and, with a full lung, bend backwards, exhaling in your maximum backwards bend for a count of 5, breathing normally. Inhale gently as you return to an upright position. Exhale, relax and repeat the entire sequence.

Help and Advice

When you first start the Rishis posture, you may find the movement is much easier on one side than the other. It is great that you have noticed this, because these imbalances can be the start of problems later on. By doing the movement, these imbalances can be carefully corrected.

Please progress at your own pace, and never feel disappointed if you are stiff. Just regard it as your starting point to a flexible, ache-free back.

The backwards bend again can prove difficult in the beginning stages, but just remember the inch rule – even if you can only move an inch backwards, that's fine; progress a tiny bit more each time you do it and you will start to feel better than you have felt for years.

7 Body Roll

This simple tension-releasing movement does wonders for your waistline while relieving lower back tension.

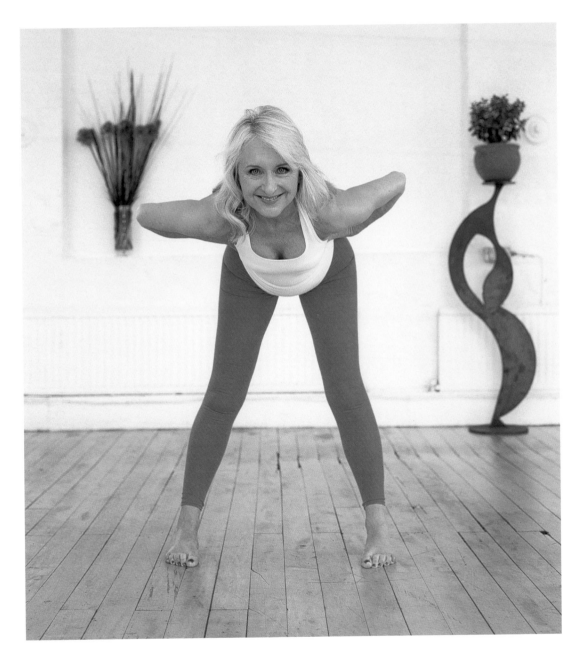

- Stand straight with your feet facing forwards and about 2 feet apart. Place your hands at your waistline with your thumbs in front and fingers behind. Inhale deeply and, as you exhale, move slowly forwards, keeping your head up.

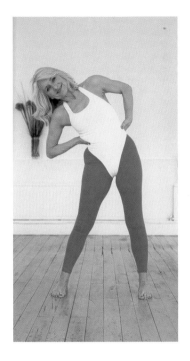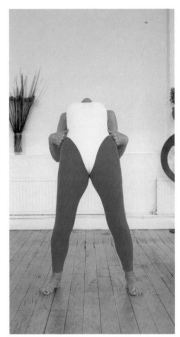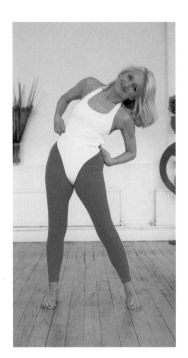

- Breathing normally, slowly and carefully, in continuous motion roll your body to the right, then carefully backwards, then to the left and slowly forwards. Do two circles to the right followed by two circles to the left. After completing the body roll, inhale deeply. Stand straight and stretch your arms straight up above your head. Place your hands together and straighten your spine. Hold the stretch for a count of 5, then exhale, slowly lower your arms and relax.

Help and Advice

The Body Roll is such a nice easy exercise – it rarely presents many problems. Just remember to start with a small circle and expand it as your flexibility improves. Always finish by stretching to realign the spine.

8   Awkward Posture

This important movement firms and tones your thighs while increasing the flexibility of your feet, knees and ankles.

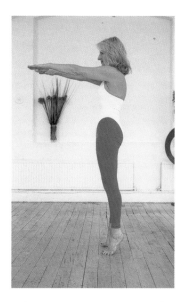 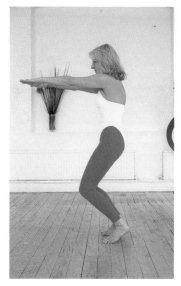 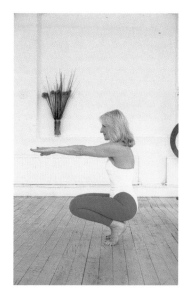

- Stand straight with your feet about a foot apart, your toes pointing forwards. Place your arms parallel to the floor. Inhale and gently come up onto your toes.

- As you exhale, keeping your back straight, slowly lower your bottom to your heels. Please don't worry if only halfway is possible to begin with, move at your own pace without strain.

- Hold your maximum position in the movement for a count of 5. Then inhale and gradually return to an upright position, keeping your back straight. Exhale, relax and repeat the movement twice.

Help and Advice
It can be very disturbing to suddenly discover that your knees, feet and ankles have stiffened up. Again, the 'use it or lose it' principle applies here. Cheer up – even if your joints are very stiff, a little practice a day does work wonders.

9 Toe Balance

This movement helps your sense of balance and concentration, and strengthens your toes and the arches of your feet.

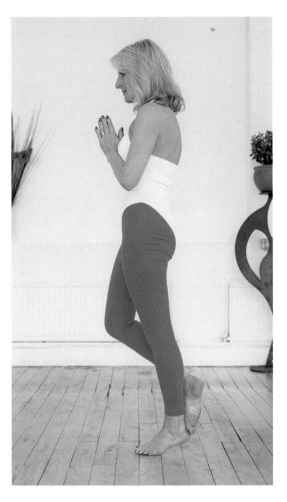

- Stand straight and place your hands as if in prayer.
- Place your right foot behind your left ankle. Breathe in and gently come up onto your toes. Exhale and hold the position, staring at a spot on the wall or floor to help you to balance for a count of 5, breathing normally.
- Lower your heels down to the floor, relax and repeat on the other side. Then repeat the entire sequence twice. Increase the hold to a count of 10 as you progress in the movement.

'I was introduced to Barbara Currie's excellent yoga classes by a good friend, at a time when I was suffering from severe stress and felt close to complete exhaustion. Now I am fit, healthy, happy, relaxed, positive and more flexible than I have been since I was a child. Thank you, Barbara.'

JOANNE, 64

Help and Advice
I know this looks so simple, yet you may find you can't do it. You wobble around or find it difficult to lift your heels from the floor. Again, this is normal. Stay calm and concentrate on that spot on the wall or floor, and gradually you will find your sense of balance and your feet strengthening.

Yoga teaches us that the mind is like the sun's rays: normally they shine on all of us and give us warmth, but concentrate them on one spot and they are powerful enough to cause fire. The mind, likewise, when it concentrates on one thing at a time, becomes extremely powerful, as all the minor thoughts and worries of daily life start to vanish and your mind becomes clear and calm.

10 Tree Balance

This position increases the flexibility of your hips, knees and ankles, tones your inner and outer thighs, strengthens your supporting leg and again helps your balance and concentration.

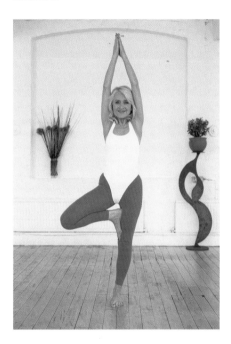

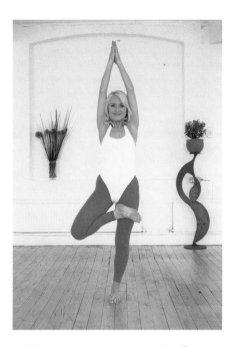

- Stand straight with perfect posture and both feet together, your hands by your sides. Breathe in as you place your right foot on your left thigh. (Choose a position to suit yourself to begin with, perhaps resting your foot on your calf or ankle. Gradually, as you improve in the movement, lift your foot higher up your leg until it is eventually resting on your upper thigh.)

- Now stare at a spot on the floor or straight in front of you (remember, this is the secret of balance) and lift your arms up above your head. Straighten your arms and your spine and hold this position for a count of 5, increasing to 10 as you improve in the position, breathing normally. Exhale slowly as you lower your arms and relax. Repeat on the other side, then repeat the entire sequence once.

Help and Advice

Stiff hips, knees and ankles and an inability to balance are the main problems here. I do promise you it is worth it! Concentrate on your spot and, even if you start by placing your foot on your ankle, that's fine. Just continue daily practice; perseverance will relieve the stiffness carefully and give you back the flexibility of youth!

15-Minute Miracles
Stage 2

This sequence will teach you the huge benefits of correct breathing. It will help to relieve tension in the neck and shoulders and correct your posture. It will do wonders for your thighs and strengthen your bones, firm and tone virtually every muscle in your body, and help your concentration.

- The Complete Breath
- Chest Expansion
- Siamese Posture
- Warrior Posture I
- Warrior Posture II
- Half-Moon Balance
- The Triangle
- Big Toe Balance
- Dancer's Posture

Health is the only thing that makes you think that now is the very best time of year.
FRANKLIN ADAMS

1   The Complete Breath

Yoga teaches us that 'Life is breath, and he who only half-breathes only half-lives.' Because deep, thorough breathing is so important to our health, looks and feeling of well-being, it is worth taking a lot of trouble with this brilliant breathing exercise. It will calm you down in times of stress, help you sleep well at night and energize your whole system. Most people breathe too quickly making inadequate use of the lungs. This breathing exercise makes full use of the lungs' tremendous oxygen-absorption capacity, leading to oxygen-rich blood.

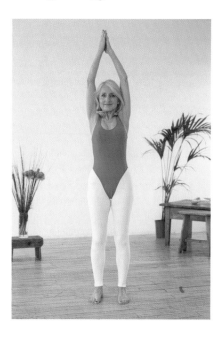

- Stand very straight with your hands by your sides and your feet about 1 foot apart. Gently push your abdominals out and inhale deeply and slowly through your nose for a count of 5, lifting your arms up above your head as you do so. Retain the breath for a count of 5.
- Slowly lower your arms as you exhale peacefully through your nose for a count of 5. At the end of your exhalation, gently, without breathing in, pull your abdominals in and up, then push them out and inhale slowly through your nose, allowing the air to fill your lungs. Hold for a count of 5, then exhale slowly and calmly for a count of 5.
- Repeat 10 times. As you become more comfortable with this exercise, gradually increase the inhalations and exhalations until you are inhaling and exhaling for a count of 10.

Help and Advice

In yoga we aim to make full use of the lungs. By pushing the abdominals out as we breathe in, we allow the diaphragm to flatten out so that we are able to fill the lungs as the ribcage expands. Retaining the breath allows for maximum oxygen absorption. The slow, calm exhalation is very controlled and very relaxing. When you lift the abdominals in and up at the end of the exhalation, you are in fact squeezing out the stale air, so that when you push the abdominals out to breathe in again you are creating negative pressure inside the chest. As nature abhors a vacuum, maximum air is brought into the lungs, so increasing the oxygen level in the blood stream.

Most people, when stressed, breathe by pulling the abdominals in as they inhale and allowing them to push out as they exhale. This does not allow for adequate oxygen absorption and can lead to low energy levels.

I really do recommend this breathing exercise, so spend some time on it, getting it right. It will be a real friend to you in times of need.

2   Chest Expansion

How do people live without this movement? It releases tension in the back, neck, shoulder and chest, firms and tones the upper arms and muscles that support the bust, stimulates blood flow to the head and neck area, firms the throat and jaw, tones the back of the thighs and calves, and gives incredible flexibility to the spine.

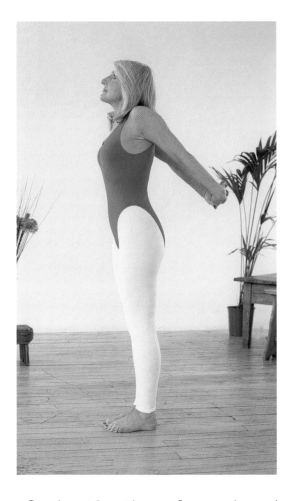 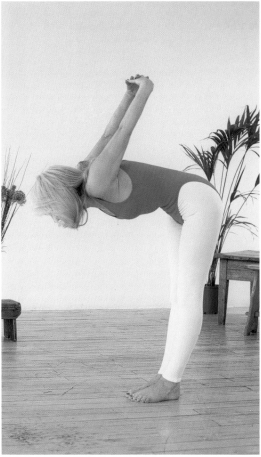

• Stand straight with your feet together and interlock your hands behind your back. Inhale and lift your arms up as high as possible, ensuring that your elbows are straight.

• Exhale slowly and, with your head up, your back flat and your legs straight, gently move forwards into your maximum forward bend.

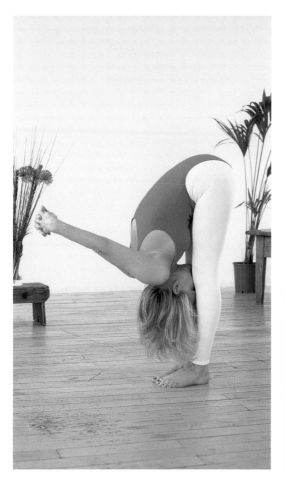

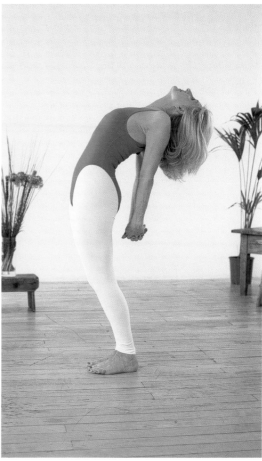

• Hold this maximum position for a count of 5, breathing normally, then inhale, lift your head and slowly return to an upright position.

• Gently relax backwards, pulling your arms downwards and exhaling in your maximum position. Hold this backwards stretch for a count of 5, breathing normally, then inhale and return to an upright position, exhale and relax. Repeat twice.

Help and Advice

When you first start this movement, even straightening your elbows when clasping your hands behind your back can be difficult – but persevere. A lot of people hold a great deal of tension in their shoulders and neck, which can contribute to headaches, migraine and many other stress-related problems. By practising this movement daily without strain, you will experience great relief from this tension and be delighted with the great shape it gives your arms!

3 Siamese Posture

This movement does wonders for your waistline and midriff, keeps your spine flexible and tones your throat and jaw.

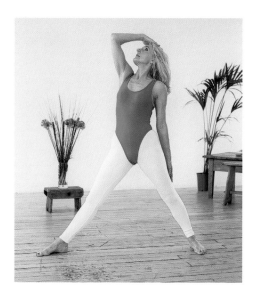

- Stand straight with your legs 3½–4 feet apart. Turn your right foot at a 90-degree angle to the right. Place your right hand on the top of your head and look at the centre of your elbow.

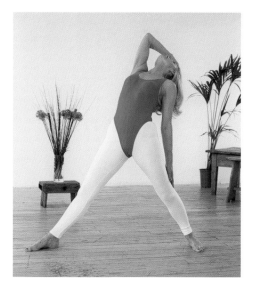

- Inhale deeply. Then, as you exhale, slide your left hand down your left leg as far as possible. Keep your gaze on the centre of your right elbow. Hold your maximum stretch for a count of 5, breathing normally, then inhale and return to an upright position, exhale and relax and repeat on the left side. Repeat the entire sequence.

'In my late fifties I had an accident which damaged my knees so badly that I could not walk or swim. I decided to try yoga, and have never looked back. Today my knees are largely recovered and I am fitter and more flexible than ever before.'

MAUREEN, 68

4   Warrior Posture I

The Warrior Posture firms and tones your thighs and releases lower back tension. It gives fantastic shape to your legs, streamlining your calves and firming your buttocks.

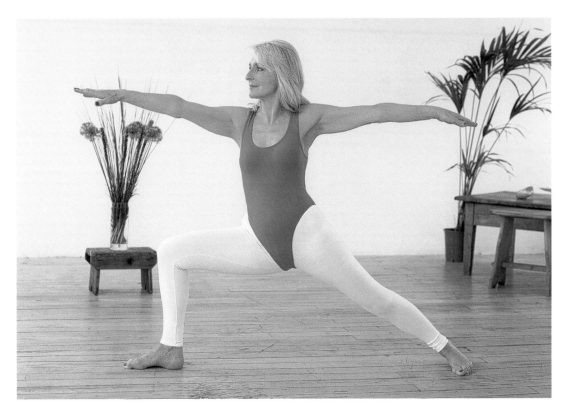

- Stand with your legs about 3½–4 feet apart and turn your right foot 90 degrees to the right, your left foot facing forwards. Stretch your arms outwards and parallel to the floor.
- Inhale deeply and, as you exhale, bend your right leg, aiming eventually to have your right thigh parallel to the floor and the left one straight. Ensure that the outer edge of your left foot stays on the floor and fix your gaze on the centre of your right hand.
- Hold your maximum stretch in this movement for a count of 5, lengthening the hold to a count of 10 as you become more adept at the movement. Inhale and return to an upright position. Exhale, relax and repeat to the other side. Repeat the entire sequence.

Help and Advice
In the beginning stages, although this movement looks easy, you may find it very difficult to keep the outer portion of your left foot on the floor. This is quite normal, and again will come with practice. Also trying to have your thigh flat and your left leg straight can be a huge problem to start with, but this pose slims and streamlines your thighs and calves and keeps them in great shape for life. I really recommend it.

5   Warrior Posture II

This movement has all the benefits of the previous posture but also relieves tightness in the chest and neck, firms and tones the jaw and throat, and corrects posture.

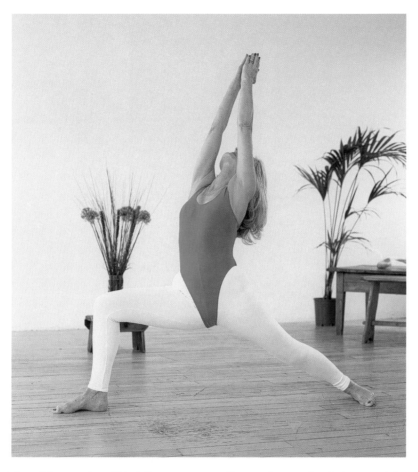

- Stand straight with your legs 3½–4 feet apart. Turn your right foot 90 degrees to the right, your left foot facing forwards. Drop your head back and stretch your arms above your head, placing them together and crossing your thumbs.
- Breathe in deeply and, as you exhale, bend your right leg, again aiming to keep your thigh flat and your back leg straight. Keep your gaze on your hands and breathe normally in your maximum position. Hold for a count of 5, increasing to 10 as you improve in the movement.
- Repeat on the other side, then repeat the entire sequence.

Help and Advice
Sometimes dropping your head back and looking at your hands is difficult, so just do your best; it is a great tension-reliever and an excellent aid to correcting poor posture.

6 Half-Moon Balance

This movement tones and firms your buttocks and thighs. It greatly increases the flexibility in your lower back, tones and strengthens your arms and helps your concentration and balance.

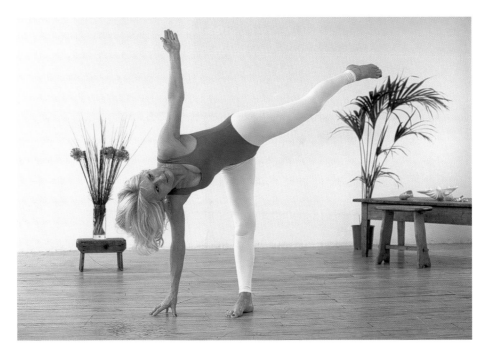

- Stand straight with your feet 1 foot apart and turn your right foot 90 degrees to the right. Concentrate on a spot on the right side of your body and stretch your right arm out to the side. Inhale deeply and, as you exhale, aim to place your right hand on the floor, bending your knees if necessary to enable you to do this.
- Now lift your left leg in the air carefully and extend your left arm, trying to keep this arm in line with your right arm. When you are comfortable in this position, gently rotate your shoulders to enable you to look up at your left hand.
- Hold this position for a count of 5 (increasing to 10 as you improve in the position), breathing normally, then exhale and lower your left arm and then your left leg. Gently come up into a standing position. Exhale and relax. Repeat on the other side, then repeat the entire sequence.

Help and Advice
If you find this very difficult in the beginning, just practise by standing straight and lifting your left leg and left arm out to the side while stretching your right arm to the right. Start by raising the leg just a little at first and then practise by leaning to the right a little as you do this. Keep practising and eventually you will have the confidence to put your right hand on the floor.

7 The Triangle

This incredible yoga sequence works virtually every muscle, tendon, joint and internal organ in the body. It tones and firms the hips, thighs, waistline and arms. It revitalizes the spine and helps correct lower back tension and stiffness.

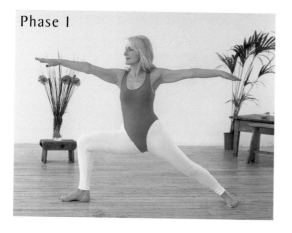

Phase 1

- Stand straight with your legs 3½–4 feet apart. Turn your right foot 90 degrees to the right. Your left foot faces forwards. Inhale and place your arms at shoulder level parallel to the floor. Exhale as you bend your right leg, aiming to keep your thigh flat and back leg straight.

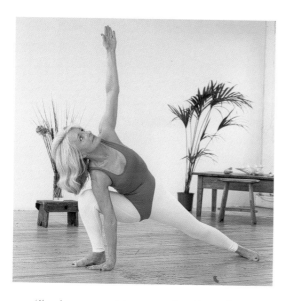

- Place your right hand by your right foot, if possible with your little finger by your big toe. If this is not possible, hold your ankle or calf. Now lift your left arm in the air and point your fingers to the ceiling. Aiming to have both arms in a straight line, ensure that the outside of your left foot remains on the floor. Turn your head to look at the ceiling, aiming your chin in line with your left shoulder. Hold this position for a count of 5, increasing to 10 as you improve in the movement, breathing normally. Inhale as you return to an upright position. Exhale and relax, then repeat to the other side.

'I've been practising yoga for about five years now. I first started doing it as a way of getting some respite from the storm of having four children! I'd found that the kind of exercise I'd done in the past – tennis, skiing, squash – only added to the adrenaline of having a busy life, so I was looking for something more calming. Yoga really grounds me and slows me down. It makes me take time out and take care of myself, which I think is really important when you're a mother and have so many other people to think about!'

RACHEL, 41

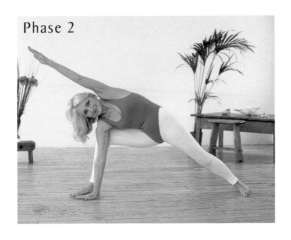

Phase 2

- Stand as above, with your legs 3½–4 feet apart and your right foot turned 90 degrees to the right, your left foot facing forwards, arms parallel to the floor at shoulder level.
- Inhale deeply and, as you exhale, bend your right knee, aiming to keep your thigh flat and back leg straight. Try to place your right little finger by your right big toe. Place your left arm alongside your left ear, in a straight line with your left foot.
- Hold for a count of 5, increasing to 10 as the movement becomes easier. Inhale and return to an upright position. Exhale and relax, then repeat to the left side.

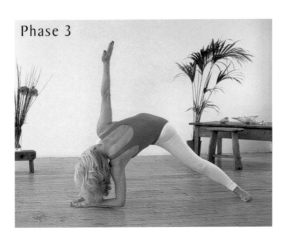

Phase 3

- With your legs 3½–4 feet apart, arms parallel to the floor, right foot at 90 degrees to the right and your left foot facing forwards, take a deep breath in and change your arms over so that your left arm faces over your right leg.
- Inhale and, bending your right leg, aim to have your thigh flat. Place your left hand by your right foot with your left thumb by your right big toe. Gently lift your right arm in the air and rotate your torso so that you are looking at your right hand. Hold for a count of 5, breathing normally, increasing to 10 as you improve in the movement, and then slowly return to an upright position.
- Exhale, lower your arms and relax. Repeat to the left side, then repeat the entire triangle sequence.

Help and Advice

Because the Triangle is such an incredibly brilliant movement it is frequently a nightmare to start with. There is no easy way to do these positions – we have all had to come to terms with our own stiffness in different regions of our bodies. All I can say is persevere, follow the directions, don't strain and eventually you will love these movements and the incredible benefits that they will give you.

8 Big Toe Balance

This posture gives you back your youth. It feels so great to be able to lift your leg higher than you could as a teenager. It does wonders for the shape of your legs, reduces cellulite, firms your bottom and thighs, releases tension in your lower back and helps your concentration.

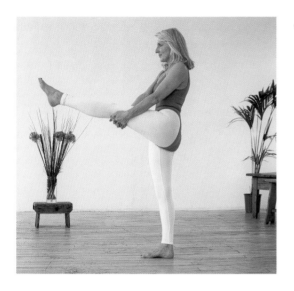

- Stand straight and place your right hand on your right hip. Concentrate on a spot for balance and clasp your left big toe in your left hand. If this is too difficult for you, just place both your hands under your left knee.

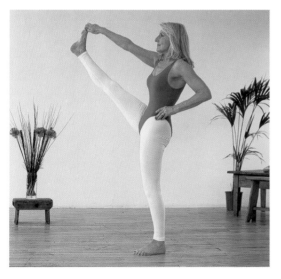

- Now, while staring at your spot and keeping your supporting leg straight, try to straighten and lift your leg. Hold this for a count of 5, increasing to 10 as you improve in the position. Exhale, lower your leg and relax. Repeat on the other side. Repeat the entire sequence.

Help and Advice
Straightening both legs can be difficult even for advanced students. Don't worry; first of all try to balance in the position even if your legs are a little bent. Progress by straightening the leg on which you are standing and finally you will lift and straighten the other leg!

9 Dancer's Posture

This lovely movement helps your posture and concentration. It releases lower back tension, tones and firms your thighs and bottom and strengthens the supporting leg.

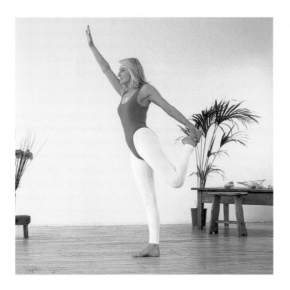

- Stand straight with perfect posture and feet together. As you inhale, lift your right arm in the air. As you exhale, grab your left foot in your left hand behind your back.

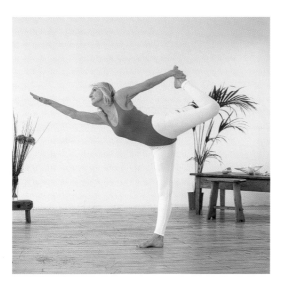

- Concentrate on a spot, inhale and, as you exhale, lean forwards and lift your left leg as high as possible, keeping your right leg straight. Hold for 5, increasing to 10 as you progress in the position. Exhale, lower your leg, relax and repeat to the other side. Repeat the entire sequence once.

Help and Advice

In the beginning stages, if you can't reach your left foot concentrate on your spot and practise balancing at first with your right arm in the air and your left leg just a few inches behind you. Hold this position and, gradually, as you improve by lifting your leg a little more each day, you will find it easier to clasp your left foot in your left hand.

15-Minute Miracles
Stage 3

This sequence will give you great energy, tone your midriff and waistline, thighs, hips and arms, strengthen your bones, give you incredible flexibility, keep spine and joint problems at bay, and firm, tone and flatten your tummy.

- Salute to the Sun
- Half-Moon Posture
- Straight Leg Triangle
- Head-to-Knee Balance
- Standing Stick Balance
- Tree Balance
- Eagle Balance
- Abdominal Lift and Contractions

The block of granite which was an obstacle in the path of the weak, becomes a stepping stone in the path of the strong.
THOMAS CARLYLE

I Salute to the Sun

This is your stay-young insurance policy. After 30 years of teaching yoga to literally thousands of pupils, I can tell you now that in my experience people who do this sequence daily for life quite simply walk younger, stand straighter, look better, are more radiant and have more energy and vitality than those who don't.

Salute to the Sun gives you energy; it stretches your body from top to toe; its brilliant combination of clever stretches and deep breathing – traditionally done facing the sunrise in the east – prepares your body to start the day.

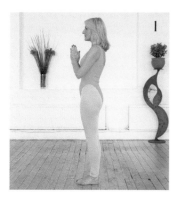

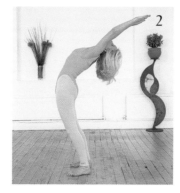

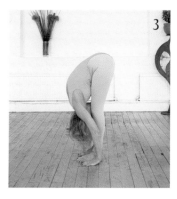

- Stand straight with your feet either about 12 inches apart or together, (for a stronger stretch). Place your hands together, as if in prayer. Inhale slowly and deeply, then slowly exhale through your nose.

- Inhale deeply and lift your arms up above your head. Keeping your eyes on your thumbs, relax and bend backwards, exhaling, into your maximum position.

- Inhaling, slowly return to an upright position, stretching your arms up in the air. Keep your head up, your back flat and legs straight and slowly bend forwards and relax in your maximum position without straining.

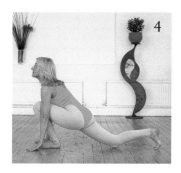

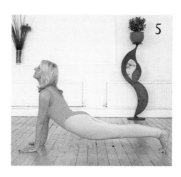

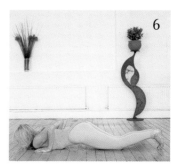

- Keeping your hands on the floor, inhale and stretch your right leg back and look at the sky.

- Exhale and stretch your left leg back.

- Now take your knees to the floor, then your chest and then your chin.

LOOK 15 YEARS YOUNGER

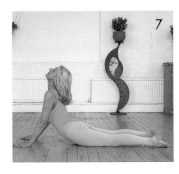

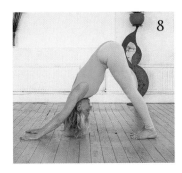

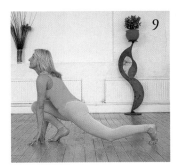

- With your lower abdomen on the floor and your hands either side of your body at shoulder level, inhale and slowly lift your upper body from the floor and stretch gently back into the Cobra position.

- Tucking in your toes, press down on your hands and lift your bottom in the air as you exhale and stretch your heels down towards the floor. Gently lower your head between your arms towards the floor.

- Inhale and draw your right foot forwards, placing it near your hands.

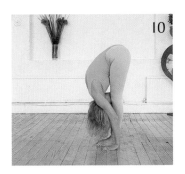

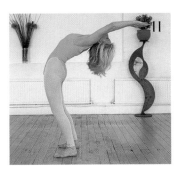

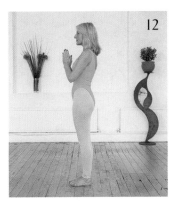

- Exhale and bring your left foot forwards. Now, drop your head and lift your bottom in the air (eventually you'll be able to touch your chin to your shins with your hands flat on the floor by your feet).

- Inhale and slowly lift your head and arms. Gently return to a standing position. With full lungs, slowly stretch upwards and then backwards, exhaling when you reach your maximum position.

- Inhale as you return to an upright position. Place your hands in prayer, exhale, relax and repeat – this time taking your left leg back first in step 5.

Help and Advice

This is a brilliant sequence, so have patience and go gently to begin with. It may take many, many weeks before it becomes a real pleasure. Sometimes it helps to do the upwards stretch and forwards and backwards bend first. Many pupils say that they are too stiff to do it first thing in the morning! Sorry, but that is why we do it. It is so easy just to accept the fact that your body becomes stiffer with age. It will if you don't stretch on waking, like every other animal on the planet does. By working at Salute to the Sun diligently on a daily basis you can keep that young spine and youthful energy for ever.

2 Half-Moon Posture

I am so grateful to this position – it has helped me maintain my 24-inch waistline so that on my 60th birthday it was the same as it was on my 18th!

It will do the same for you: It will whittle your waistline, remove your spare tyre and tone up your midriff, both front and back, and keep your spine tremendously flexible.

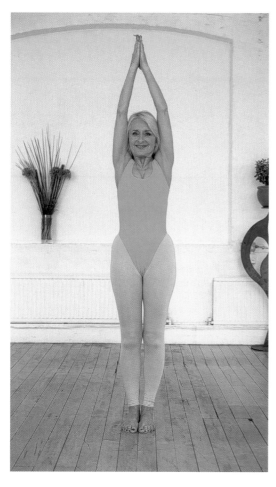

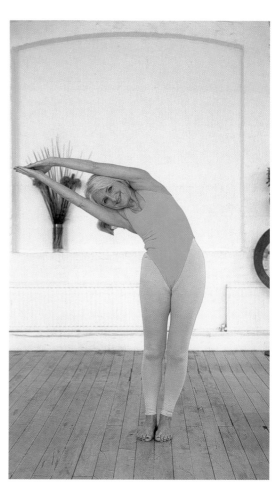

- Stand straight with your feet together. Inhale and lift your arms in the air, placing your palms together and crossing your thumbs. Stretch your arms upwards, straightening them so that the insides of your upper arms are on your ears.

- As you exhale, move slowly to the right, pushing your hips a little to the left. Keep your body in line – don't move forwards or backwards. Hold for a count of 5 breathing normally, then slowly inhale and return to an upright position. Exhale as you move, to the left, pushing your hips to the right. Hold for a count of 5, then inhale and return to an upright position.

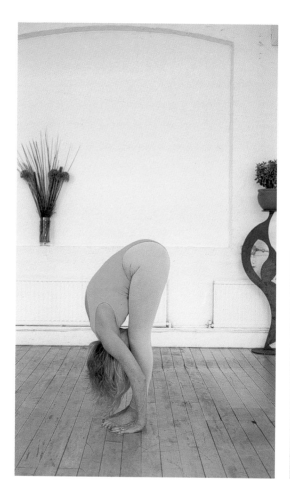 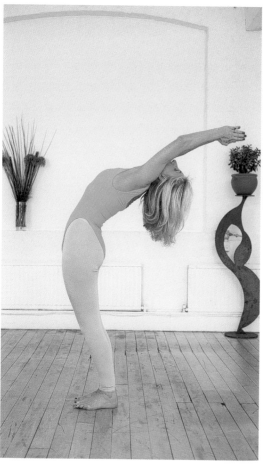

- Exhale and bend forwards with your head up, keeping your back flat and your legs straight. Relax in your maximum forwards bend without strain (eventually your aim is to be able to place your hands by your feet and your chin on your shins). Hold your maximum position for a count of 5 breathing normally.

- Inhale slowly, lift your head and arms, and gently return to an upright position. Stretch your arms up above your head. Now, concentrating on your thumbs, gently bend backwards with a full lung. Exhale in your maximum backwards bend and hold your maximum movement for a count of 5. Inhale and return to an upright position. Exhale, relax and repeat.

Help and Advice

Doesn't it look simple! Even standing straight with your head between your arms can be quite a challenge. Please just go at your own pace – if you can only move a little from side to side and forwards and back to start with, that is fine. You will still benefit and, as you start to do the movement on a regular basis, your waist measurement will show you that it is working!

3 Straight Leg Triangle

The Triangle works the entire body, toning the spinal nerves, firming and toning all the muscles around the abdomen, midriff, waistline, legs, arms and shoulders. It rids your spine of tension and gives it tremendous flexibility. This movement is excellent for the lower back and can help relieve lower backache. The backwards bend relieves tightness in the chest and tones the throat and jaw.

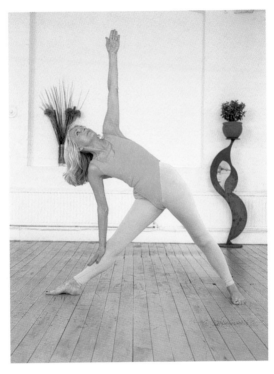

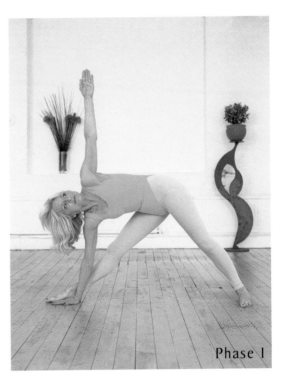

Phase 1

- Stand straight with your legs about 3½–4 feet apart.
- Turn your right foot 90 degrees to the right, keeping your left foot facing forwards. Stretch your arms outwards at shoulder level, parallel to the floor: make sure that your legs stay straight throughout this movement.

- Inhale and, facing over your right leg, exhale and slowly lower your right hand to the floor, aiming to place your right hand by your right foot with your little finger by your big toe. If this is not possible, don't bend your knee – simply hold your knee, calf or ankle. Now gently pull your left shoulder back, lift your left arm in the air and, keeping both arms in a straight line, gently look at your left hand.
- Hold this movement for a count of 5, increasing to 10 as you progress in the posture.
- Inhale as you return to an upright position. Exhale and relax. Repeat to the left side.

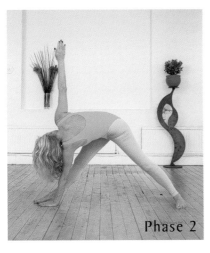

Phase 2

- With your feet about 3½–4 feet apart and your arms parallel to the floor, inhale and change your arms over so that your left hand faces over your right foot. Exhale and, keeping your legs straight, aim to place your left thumb by your right big toe – again, if this is not possible simply hold your knee, ankle or calf. Lift your right arm in the air.
- Carefully rotate your trunk so that you are gazing at your right hand. Aim to have both arms in line with each other. Hold your maximum position in this movement for a count of 5, increasing to 10 as you progress.
- Inhale and lift your left arm from the floor, then carefully return to an upright position. Exhale, relax and repeat on the other side. Repeat the entire movement once.

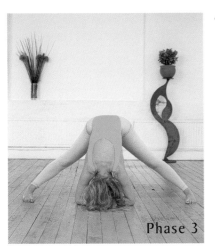

Phase 3

- With your legs 3½–4 feet apart, stand straight and ensure that your toes face forwards. Inhale and stretch both arms up in the air. Keeping your back flat and your legs straight, exhale and relax gently forwards into your maximum position. Just let go in this stretch – you will find that just by relaxing into it you are able to move further into the posture. Eventually you will be able to fold your arms and place your elbows on the floor, resting your head on your arms. In the meantime, just enjoy the movement and place your hands on your legs in your maximum stretch. Hold your best position for a count of 5, increasing to 10 as you improve. Carefully draw your feet inwards until they are only 3 feet apart.

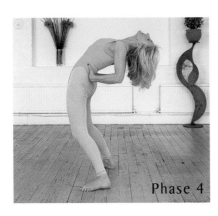

Phase 4

- Inhale and, lifting your head first, slowly return to an upright position and stretch your arms up above your head. Exhale and relax. Place your hands at your waistline with your fingers behind and thumbs in front. Now inhale deeply and gently bend backwards. Exhale in your maximum position and hold your backwards bend for a count of 5, increasing gradually to 10 as you progress. Inhale and slowly return to an upright position. Exhale and relax.

Help and Advice

This movement frequently shows up your stiff areas. The most important point is to go carefully, at your own pace, and RELAX in your maximum movement. This way your stiffness will be gently eased and the movement will help you to wonderful flexibility.

4 Head-to-Knee Balance

This is a fantastic toner for the back of your thighs and calves. It helps to reduce cellulite. It strengthens your sense of balance and your supporting leg, stretches your hamstrings and releases lower back tension.

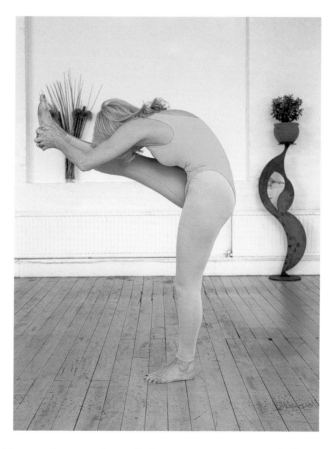

- Stand straight with your feet together, inhale and clasp your right foot with both hands. Stare at a spot on the floor for balance. Gently stretch your right leg and aim your chin towards your right knee.
- Aim to straighten your right leg, keeping your supporting (left) leg really straight. Hold your maximum stretch for 5, again increasing to 10 as you improve in the movement.
- Gently lower your leg to the floor, relax and repeat on the other side. Repeat the entire sequence.

Help and Advice
This really makes you concentrate! Please don't worry if in the beginning you can't straighten your leg. Try to keep your supporting leg straight, and remember that daily practice will enable you to do the movement.

5 Standing Stick Balance

This beautiful movement streamlines your body. It will firm and tone your bottom, thighs and calves and also strengthen them tremendously. It will tone and firm your upper arms and shoulders and is a fantastic tension-release for your entire body.

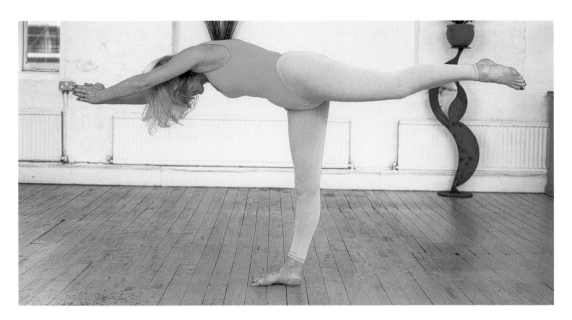

- Stand straight with your feet together and your arms up above your head, hands together and thumbs crossed. Inhale deeply and place your right foot 3 feet in front of your left one. Concentrate on a spot to enable you to balance.
- As you exhale, gently stretch forwards placing your weight on your right leg and lifting your left leg from the floor. Keep stretching forwards so that your arms are parallel to the floor and your head stays between your arms. With your left leg lifted from the floor and parallel to the floor, your entire body is stretched and resembles a capital 'T'. Hold this position for a count of 5, breathing normally and stretching while in the position. Increase the hold to 10 as your strength increases.
- Inhale and slowly lower your left leg to the floor, placing your feet together. Gently lift your arms up above your head and stretch your entire body upwards in a perfect straight line from top to toe. Relax and repeat on the other side, then repeat the entire balance.

Help and Advice
At first it isn't even easy to stand straight with your head between your straight arms and your hands together, thumbs crossed. Doing this, however, and concentrating on your posture in this position makes such a difference. Try doing it in front of a full-length mirror and you will see your imbalances. Cheer up, though; daily practice of this movement will do wonders to correct your posture. In the movement it is hard trying to make the arms and legs level, but this will become very easy as you learn to juxtapose your body in the movement.

6 Tree Balance

We first tried the tree balance in Stage 1 (page 16). Now it is time to try the entire Tree Balance. This movement does wonders for the joints in your legs; it literally oils your hips, knees, ankles and feet. It tones and firms all the muscles in your legs and is excellent for helping to prevent arthritis and rheumatism in your joints. It also helps your powers of concentration, balance and patience.

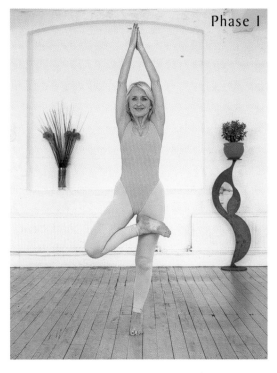

Phase 1

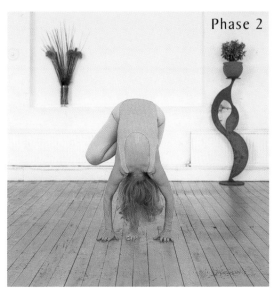

Phase 2

- Stand straight with your feet together, then lift your right foot onto your left thigh (if this is still difficult for you, just place your foot in a comfortable position, as explained in Stage 1.) Don't progress onto Phase 2 or 3 until you have mastered this position.
- Staring at a spot to enable you to balance, inhale and lift your arms straight up in the air, placing your palms together and crossing your thumbs. Hold this position for a count of 5, increasing to 10 as your strength improves.
- Exhale, lower your arms and leg, place your hands together and relax. Repeat on the other side, then repeat the entire movement.

- Stand with your right foot on your left thigh and your arms straight above your head as in Phase 1.
- Inhale and, as you exhale, staring at a spot on the floor, gently move forwards, aiming to place your hands on the floor either side of your left foot and, eventually, your chin on your shin. (This is rarely possible in the beginning stages.) Move only as far as you can without strain – this at first may be just a few inches, which is fine.
- Relax in your maximum position, breathing normally for a count of 5, then find another spot and concentrate hard on it, and then slowly lift first your head and then your upper body and eventually return to an upright standing position. Lower your leg and arms and relax. Repeat on the other side.

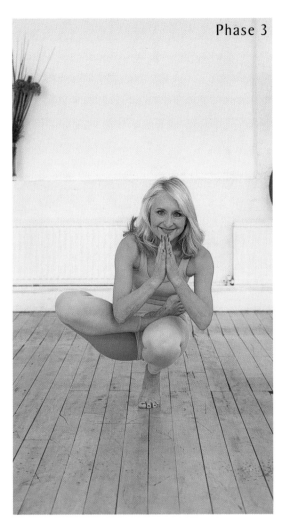

Phase 3

(Only move into this phase when you can easily manage Phase 2.)

- Stand straight with your right foot on your left thigh and place your arms above your head, palms together. Inhale and, as you exhale, carefully move forwards and place your hands flat on the floor by your left foot as in Phase 2.

- Now place your hands about 2 feet in front of your feet and transfer the majority of your weight to your hands, coming onto the ball of your left foot. Concentrate on a spot and gently lower your bottom to balance on your left heel. Now adjust your posture so that you are literally sitting on your left heel. Keep concentrating on your spot and, finally, place your hands in prayer. Stay in this position for a count of 5, breathing normally.

- Place your hands back on the floor in front of you and transfer the majority of your weight to them. Lift your bottom in the air by straightening your legs, and return to an upright position. Place your hands in prayer and hold for a count of 5, then gently lower your right leg to the floor and relax. Repeat on the other side.

  Well done! There is no need to repeat this sequence.

Help and Advice

Where do I start? I think by saying that I have honestly seen this position perform miracles. At first it is literally a nightmare – nothing seems to work and you wonder if it is worth persevering, but having taught so many people for so long I have seen many tired people with painful knees and hips change into energized people free from their normal ageing aches, pains and stiffness. Please try it, but take care, practise at your pace and without pain or strain, and you'll see that it helps to keep your legs and joints in excellent condition for life. I would hate to grow old without yoga's magical movements.

'I started yoga while having chemotherapy. I had always been fit, but felt I needed something less aerobic and which promoted caring for body and mind rather than challenging them. Now that I am working again, daily yoga allows me to stay in touch with myself and focus on staying well.'

JENNY, 48

7   Eagle Balance

Another of yoga's gems, and again a brilliant movement to keep your shoulders, elbows, wrists, fingers, hips, knees, ankles and feet flexible and free from aches, pains and stiffness. It will tone your calves, thighs, hips and upper arms, and stimulate blood flow to the lower abdomen.

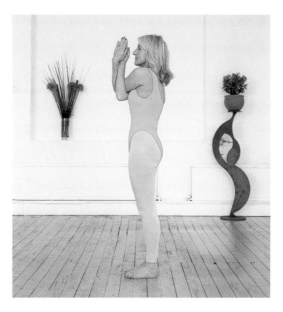

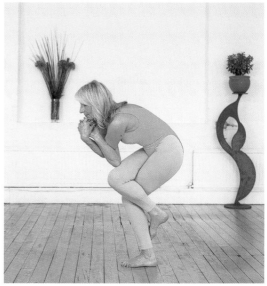

• Stand straight with both feet together. Place both arms straight out in front of you, then cross your right upper arm over your left. Take your right arm underneath the left and place your hands in prayer, with your thumbs towards you.

• Concentrate on a spot. Now take your right thigh over your left and slide your right foot behind your left calf, aiming to get all 5 toes to appear on the right side of the left calf. Now place your chin on your upper hand, your elbow on your upper knee, and a smile on your upper lip! Balance, breathing normally, for a count of 5, increasing to 10 as you progress in this position. Inhale, unwind your legs, then your arms, exhale and relax. Repeat to the other side.

Help and Advice
Try to do the arm movement first, concentrating on your spot. Then try with the legs. Remember, just a small amount of each movement will be fine to begin with. It is always a nasty shock to realize how stiff some of our joints have become. It is, however, always possible to help stiff and aching joints. Persevere and this movement will work wonders!

8 Abdominal Lift and Contractions

When I think of all the movements in yoga, these are the ones most practised and loved by my pupils. I regard them as a wonderful gift. The Lift will give you a firm, flat, beautifully-toned tummy and will prevent the abdominal drop that so often can occur with age. The Contractions relieve tension in the lower abdomen and massage the small intestine, colon, pancreas, heart and gall bladder. These movements can be most helpful to those suffering from bloating, constipation and irritable bowel syndrome. They must be done on an empty stomach – by far the best time to do them is before breakfast.

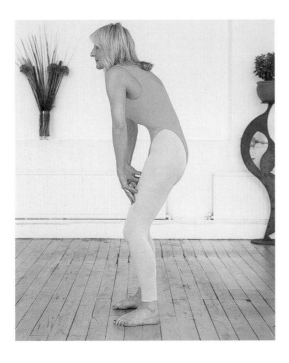

ABDOMINAL LIFT

- Stand straight with your legs about 1 foot apart and place your hands on your upper thighs. Inhale very deeply, then exhale fully.
- Keeping the air out of your lungs, pull your abdominals in and up. Hold for a count of 10, then release the abdominals. Inhale and relax. Repeat twice.

ABDOMINAL CONTRACTIONS

- With your legs about 1 foot apart, inhale deeply and then exhale. Keeping the air out of your lungs, lean slightly forwards, rest your hands on your upper thighs and snap your abdominals in and out 10 times.
- Relax and inhale. Repeat twice.

'I fell off a horse when I was 19. My hips have always been a problem, causing a twist with one leg nearly an inch different in length. I have done these classes for approximately two years and my legs are even and I feel much better.'

CATHY, 46

Help and Advice

When you first try to pull your abdominals in and up, not a lot happens. Just persevere and soon you will be in control and the firm, flat yoga tummy will soon be yours. Your mind affects every cell in your body, and during stressful times most of us have experienced the dreaded knot in our lower abdomen. We are experiencing a 'gut reaction'. The Contractions can really help to release this resulting tension.

Now you have learned your morning stretches, enjoy and make use of each day. The Romans said Carpe Diem *or 'Seize the day.' The Indian dramatist Kalidasa put it this way, in his beautiful poem that has been translated from the Sanskrit:*

Salutation to the Dawn by Kalidasa

Look to this day!

For it is life, the very life of life

In its brief course lie all the verities and realities of your existence.

The bliss of growth

The glory of action

The splendour of beauty

For yesterday is but a dream

And tomorrow is only a vision

But today well lived makes yesterday a dream of happiness

And every tomorrow a vision of hope

Look well therefore to this day

Such is the salutation to the dawn.

It is so easy to waste our precious days worrying about mistakes that we made yesterday and having anxiety over what may happen tomorrow.

Yoga teaches us to enjoy the day and live well and enjoy each moment. Worry will do you no good at all and is very, very ageing.

15-Minute Miracles
Stage 4

This beautiful relaxing sequence is an ideal aid to deep restful sleep, or indeed anytime you want to feel relaxed and calm. It will tone and stretch out your hamstrings and calves, keep your joints oiled and flexible, relieve tension in your spine and help to prevent lower back ache. It will also firm and tone your arms, calves, thighs, bottom, midriff and waistline. Above all, it will teach you to relax.

- Pose of a Heron
- Alternate Leg Pull
- Thigh Stretch
- Pose of a Star
- Simple Twist
- Backstretch
- Pose of a Cat
- Pose of a Cobra
- Half-Locust
- Full-Locust
- The Bow
- Deep Relaxation

Listen in deep silence, be very still and open your mind. Sink deep into the peace that waits for you beyond the riotous thoughts and sights and frantic sounds of this insane world.

FROM *A COURSE IN MIRACLES*

1 Pose of a Heron

This clever movement tones the backs of your thighs and is a great help in smoothing away cellulite. It stretches out your hamstrings and is a very important component in helping to relieve lower back problems.

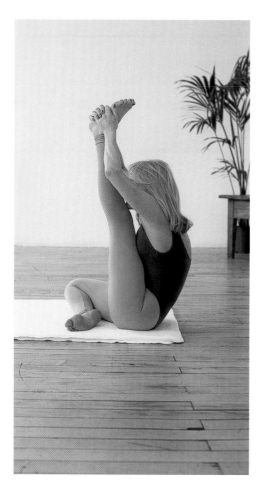

- Sit on the floor with both legs straight out in front of you. Bring your right foot into the space between your legs, resting your heel on the floor by your groin.
- Bend your left leg and interlock your hands under your left foot. Correct your posture, inhale deeply and, as you exhale, slowly aim to stretch your left leg and bring it upwards. Your eventual aim is to straighten your left leg and place your chin on your left knee, with your back and left leg straight. If this is not possible (and it rarely is in the beginning stages) simply aim to straighten your left leg – adjusting the position of your hands to your calf or knee to enable you to do this – and then lifting the leg as high as possible.
- Hold for a count of 5, breathing normally, then exhale, gently lower your leg, relax and repeat on the other side. Repeat the entire movement.

Help and Advice

Please don't worry if your hamstrings are impossibly tight in the beginning stages; this is frequently the case. However, it is essential to carefully and daily stretch them out. If you have tight hamstrings this can have the effect of putting your lumbar spine under pressure and literally making the area an accident waiting to happen. When the hamstrings are stretched this can help to ease the problem, and in my opinion stretching out the hamstrings is one of the most important factors in helping to prevent lower back problems.

2　Alternate Leg Pull

One of yoga's all-time greats! This movement ensures the flexibility of your feet, ankles, hips and thighs. It stretches and tones your hamstrings and calf muscles, rebalances your lower back and massages your lower abdominal organs.

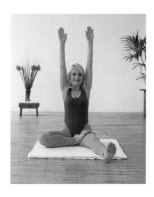

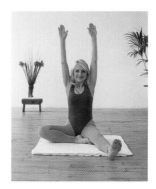

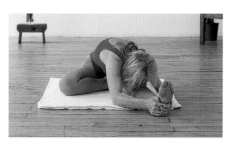

- Sit straight with both legs straight out in front of you. Carefully lift your right foot onto your left thigh. Place your right hand onto your right knee.

- Very gently and carefully bounce your knee towards the floor about six times. This movement will help you loosen your hip, knee and ankle. If your foot is comfortable on your thigh and your right knee is on the floor, then leave it there. If it isn't comfortable, just place your right foot in the space between your legs with your heel in your groin. Inhale and lift both your arms in the air.

- Exhale and, with your head up and back flat, bend forwards into your maximum position without strain. (Your eventual aim is to clasp your left foot and place your chin on your shin but, as always, whatever your maximum position in the movement is fine). Hold your maximum stretch for a count of 5, increasing to 10 as you progress in this position. Then inhale and slowly lift your head and arms and return to an upright position. Exhale and relax. Repeat the movement. Repeat on the other side, this time bringing your left foot onto your right thigh and notice any imbalances in your body. Is one side easier than the other? Is one hip stiffer than the other? It is very important to notice these imbalances and carefully correct them, or they can lead to problems in later life.

Help and Advice

This movement can be a real eye-opener. Frequently your joints are stiffer than you think, and one side of your body is very much easier than the other. These imbalances may be due to a number of things, from poor posture to imbalanced sports such as tennis or golf, which use one side of the body more than the other.

However imbalanced or stiff you are, yoga can really help correct things for you. Just practise daily and see the difference.

3   Thigh Stretch

This movement really helps to keep the flexibility of the hip joints, and tones and firms the inner thighs.

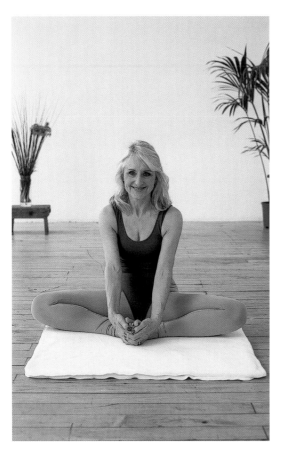

- Sit up straight and bring both your feet into the space between your legs. Place the soles of your feet together and interlock your hands around your toes.
- Take a deep breath in and, as you exhale, gently draw your knees towards the floor. Hold your maximum stretch without straining and breathe normally for a count of 5, increasing to 10 as you progress in the movement.
- Inhale as you return your knees to an upright position. Exhale, relax and repeat 3 times.

Help and Advice
This movement is so good for the health of the pelvic floor and flexibility of the hips. I can't recommend it too highly. It is an excellent movement to practise during pregnancy and really helps with the baby's delivery.

Please don't worry if at first your knees are nowhere near the floor in this position. Just practise and you'll soon see the difference.

4   Pose of a Star

A wonderful movement for releasing lower back tension, increasing the flexibility of the hips and promoting the health of the pelvic floor region. It is excellent for toning and firming the inner thighs.

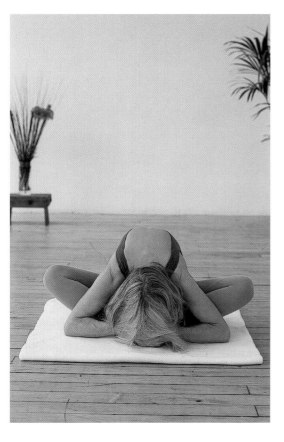

- Sit straight with both hands around the soles of your feet and draw your feet towards your groin.
- Inhale deeply and, as you exhale, gently draw your knees towards the floor and then bend forwards into your maximum position without strain, eventually aiming to get your chin to your toes.
- Breathing normally, hold your maximum position in this movement for a count of 5, increasing to 10 as you progress in it. Inhale and slowly return to an upright position, exhale, relax and repeat twice.

15-MINUTE MIRACLES – STAGE 4

Help and Advice
It is normal not to move far in this movement in the beginning stages; the hips are stiff and bending forwards can be quite difficult. Please remember, though, that you benefit at every stage in every yoga posture, and with practice you will reach your goal. It feels so good when you do – time to celebrate.

'I have a scoliosis curve in my spine. I discovered yoga four years ago, when I had terrible back pain after childbirth. Practising yoga two to three times a week keeps my back free of any pain.'
VICTORIA, 35

5 Simple Twist

This gives great strength and flexibility to your spine while toning and firming your midriff, waistline and hips. The movement massages your internal organs, stimulating the circulation to the kidneys, liver and spleen.

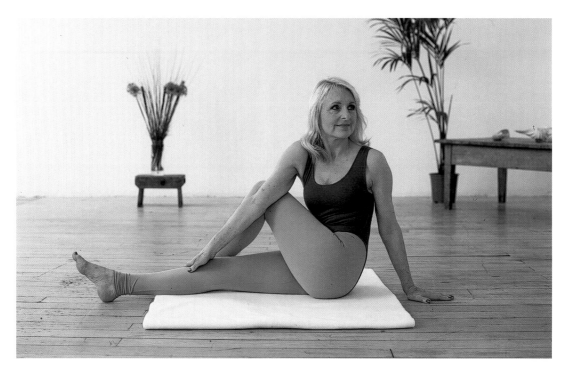

- Sit straight with both legs straight out in front of you. Lift your left leg over your right and place it on the floor on the outside of your right thigh.
- Inhale and place your left hand on the floor behind your back, then take your right arm to the outside of your left knee and place it on your right knee. Exhale slowly and, with perfect posture, rotate your torso to the left and turn your head over your left shoulder.
- Hold your maximum stretch in this position for a count of 5, increasing to 10 as you progress in the movement. Slowly return your head to the front and repeat. Perform the movement twice on the other side.

Help and Advice
Sometimes it is not possible to take the right hand to the right knee in the beginning stage, so just let it rest in your maximum position. If twisting is difficult, again don't push or strain, just do your best and with practice you will get there. You will start to really experience the benefits of the twist when you next park your car!

6 Backstretch

Following the Simple Twist, it is essential to realign your spine – the Backstretch is the perfect movement for this. It releases lower back tension, firms and tones your abdominal area, stretches your spine, hamstrings and calves, and massages your heart.

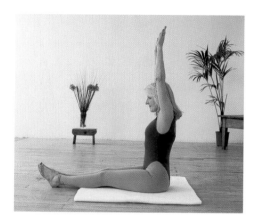

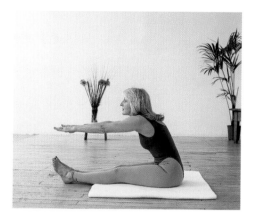

- Sit straight with both legs straight out in front of you. Inhale deeply and lift both your arms straight up in the air.

- Exhale as you slowly bend forwards with your head up and back flat into your own maximum position without strain.

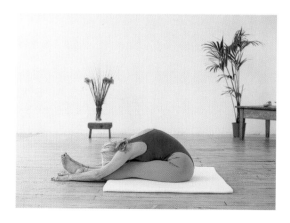

- Remember, only a little way to begin with is fine. Your eventual aim, however, is to be able to clasp your ankles and place your chin on your shins. Stay in your maximum position, breathing normally, for a count of 5, increasing to 10 as you progress in the movement. Inhale, lift your head and arms and slowly and carefully return to an upright position. Exhale, lower your arms and relax. Repeat twice.

Help and Advice

This is a yoga essential, but due to many factors – from tight hamstrings and stiff hips to a rigid lumbar spine – it can be difficult in the initial stages. However, the earlier movements in this Stage will greatly help you to achieve rapid progress in the backstretch and help to rejuvenate your entire spine.

7 Pose of a Cat

Watch a cat wake up and carefully stretch his spine from top to bottom by moving each vertebra in turn. This ensures that his spine is tension-free and ready for action. Oh, if only the human race did the same!

By practising the Cat stretch you too can release tension from your spine and really help an aching back. The movement will also tone and firm your jaw, throat, bottom, thighs and your upper arms, and strengthen your wrists and hands.

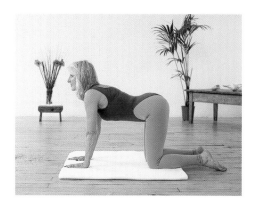

Phase 1

- In an all-fours position, ensure that your hands and knees are about 1 foot apart.

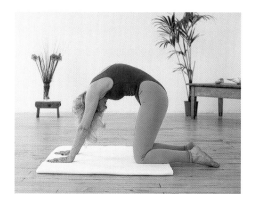

- Inhale deeply and arch your body like a cat in a bad mood, dropping your head between your arms.

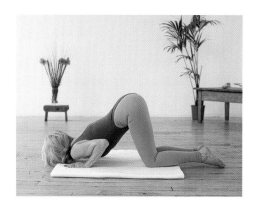

- Exhale as you lift your head and look at the ceiling, at the same time lowering your back so that your bottom sticks out. Repeat the above sequence in a slow, continuous motion 5 times. This alone can relieve tension and help an aching back.

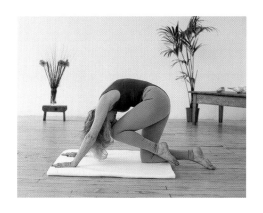

Phase 2

- In an all-fours position as in Phase 1, now bend your elbows and place your chin on the floor. Inhale and again arch your back into a hump and gently draw your right knee to your forehead.

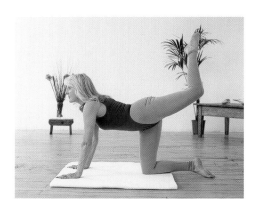

- Exhale, lift your head and look at the ceiling, lifting your right leg in the air and pointing your toes to the ceiling. Repeat the above sequence 3 times, then repeat with the left leg.

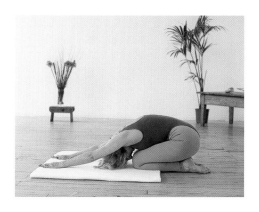

- Following the repetition, take a deep breath in and, as you exhale, gently lower your bottom to your heels, placing your forehead on the floor in front of your knees, keeping your arms at full stretch. This is called the Pose of a Swan. Stay in this position for a count of 10, breathing normally. Inhale and slowly return to an upright position, stretching your arms up above your head in a straight line with your palms together and thumbs crossed. Exhale and relax. There is no need to repeat the movement.

Help and Advice

If you find Phase 2 difficult in the beginning, don't worry. Just do Phase 1 followed by the Pose of a Swan until you feel more agile. If you do have an aching back you will find Phase 1 a real blessing. Use it after you have finished occupations that can lead to an aching back, such as gardening.

8   Pose of a Cobra

This is so relaxing, and ideal for before bedtime. It tones and strengthens your upper arms, wrists and hands, gives the spine tremendous flexibility and helps correct poor posture. It is excellent for helping to relieve menstrual cramps and backache. It tones the liver, spleen and kidneys, and stimulates the thyroid gland in the neck.

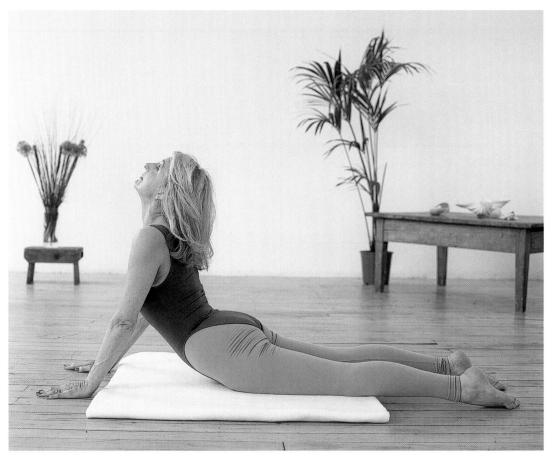

- Lie on your mat face-down with your feet together and your forehead on the floor. Your hands should be 3 inches from your body, with your fingers facing forwards and in line with your shoulders. Inhale deeply and, as you exhale, lift your head and place your chin on the floor.

- Inhale again and, keeping your lower abdominals on the floor, lift your head and upper body slowly from the floor into your maximum stretch without strain. Drop your head back and exhale in your maximum position. Again, please don't worry if only a little movement is possible in the beginning stages. Hold your maximum position for a count of 5, breathing normally, increasing the hold to a count of 10 as your strength increases.

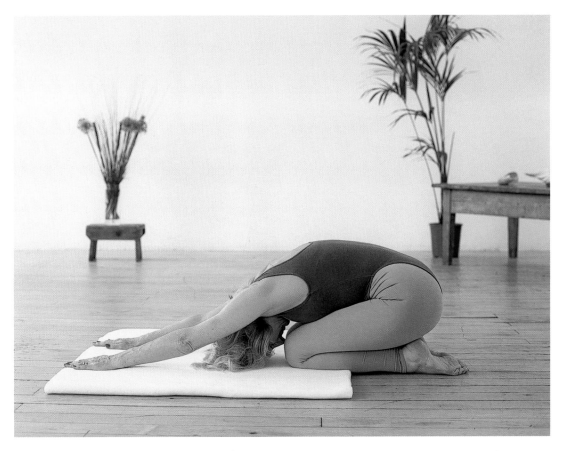

• Slowly lower yourself to the floor, place your forehead on the floor, then turn your head on one side and relax. Repeat twice. Finish by inhaling and lifting your bottom in the air; exhale and stretch back onto your heels, keeping your arms at full stretch. Relax in this position, called the Pose of a Swan, for a count of 5. Inhale and return to a kneeling position, stretch your arms up in the air, crossing your thumbs, hold for 5, then lower them, exhaling. Relax.

Help and Advice

This beautiful backwards curve of the body can be very difficult in the beginning stages but it is bound to be because in virtually everything we do in life we are curving slightly forwards. Without yoga's brilliant backwards bends this can easily lead to that ageing stoop. The Cobra will become easier very quickly; progress at your own pace without strain. If it is very difficult for you at first, simply rest on your lower arms and elbows until your back feels better, then just progress at your own pace. Soon you won't be able to live without it!

9 Half-Locust

Please do not attempt if you are pregnant

The Half-Locust relieves lower back tension and firms and tones the bottom and thighs. It releases tension in the lower abdomen and can help to relieve constipation.

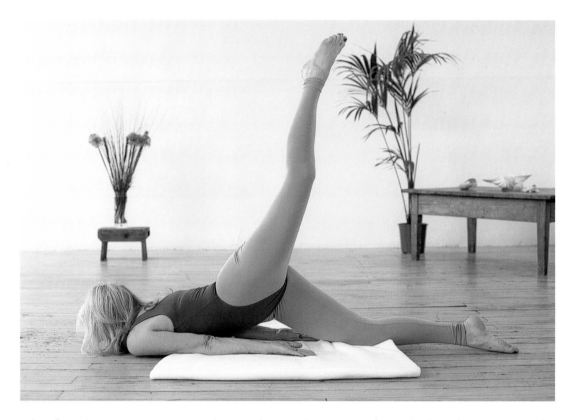

- Lie face down on your mat with your feet together and your chin on the floor. Have your hands and arms by your sides or under your thighs.
- Inhale deeply and, as you exhale, gently lift your right leg from the floor, keeping it straight. Don't twist or roll over onto your side. Hold for a count of 5, breathing normally, increasing the hold to 10 as you progress in the position.

- Lower your leg and relax, then repeat on the other side. Repeat the entire sequence twice. Lift your bottom in the air and stretch it back to your heels with your arms straight out in front of you into the Pose of a Swan. Hold for a count of 10, then gently return to an upright position.

Help and Advice

The chief problem here is that with your desire to lift your leg higher there is a tendency to roll over to the side or bend the leg. It is much better to lift the leg just a little way to begin with rather than to get into the lop-sided habit. Remember, practice makes perfect.

10 Full Locust

This posture is a wonderful strengthener for the lower back. It tones the bottom and thighs, helps to relieve constipation and menstrual troubles and can help to relieve the pain of tennis elbow. I also heartily recommend doing three of these before bed as an aid to calm, restful sleep.

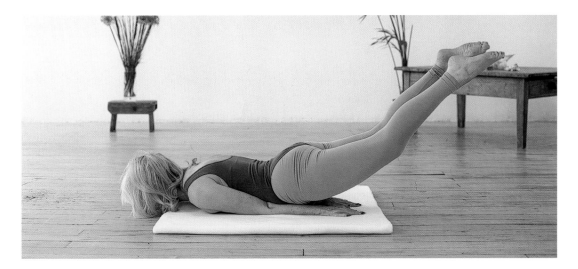

- Lie on your stomach with your chin on the floor and your arms under your body, palms facing downwards. Inhale deeply. As you exhale, lift both legs from the floor, making sure you keep them together and straight. Hold for a count of 5, then slowly lower your legs, relax and repeat twice.

- After completing the Locust posture, place your hands either side at shoulder level, inhale deeply and lift your bottom in the air and stretch it gently back to your heels and remain in this posture, known as Pose of a Swan, for a count of 5. This is an excellent movement to stretch out and realign the spine following the Locust position.

Help and Advice
Please note if you have a weak lower back please ensure that you practise the Half-Locust and feel really comfortable with it before starting the Full Locust, and then progress with caution, holding only for a count of 1 to start with, increasing to 5 as you make progress in the position.

'I first started doing yoga about 10 years ago. I was looking for something that would get my body as agile as my mind. I'd tried all sorts of things before that, such as step classes, aerobics and so on, but I didn't really feel a great benefit from it. I actually found that I came out of those kinds of classes feeling more wound-up and with less energy than when I started. With yoga, I feel much more energized, as well as calmer.'

NICKY, 48

11   The Bow

This is so relaxing, ideal to do at the end of your day. It keeps your whole body young and flexible, corrects poor posture, massages the abdominal organs and is a great help to relieve menstrual cramps. It tones the thighs, arms, throat and jaw, strengthens the abdominal muscles and can help to relieve digestive troubles.

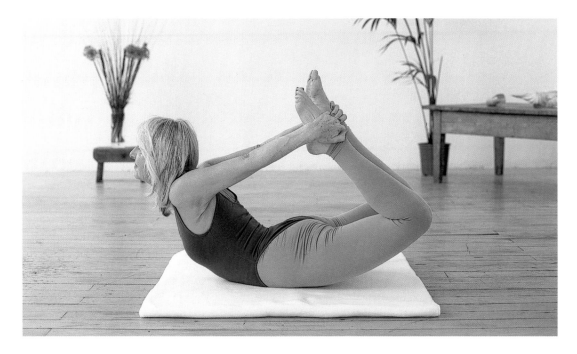

- Lie face down on your mat with your chin on the floor. Take a deep breath in and aim to clasp the outside of your feet in your hands. If this is too difficult, just stretch your arms back as far as you can without strain and, if possible, grab hold of your leggings, exhale and relax.
- Inhale again and now, holding your feet, aim to lift your head and feet as high as possible from the floor. Exhale and stay in your maximum position, breathing normally, for a count of 5, increasing to 10 as you progress in the movement. Exhale and slowly lower your body to the floor, turn your head to one side and relax. Repeat once.
- Only when you find the Bow nice and easy in your maximum position, aim to rock forwards and backwards about 2 to 3 times to begin with, then gently lower your body to the floor, place your head on one side, relax and do not repeat the rocking movement.

Help and Advice
This is a beautiful movement, but it is not easy to begin with. It will, however, give you an amazing feeling of relaxation even in the beginning stages, and with practice it makes you feel great!

12 Deep Relaxation

This is the most difficult thing to teach the average pupil, who feels that he or she is too busy to relax. This feeling of non-stop action and pressure can lead to chronic tension, which literally strangles the body, inhibiting the flow of blood and lymph to our tissues. This can lead to weakness, and eventually disease can result. Yoga exercises systematically go through the entire body, carefully stretching out the tension within, and this – along with the slow, deep breathing in every position – results in a lovely feeling of calm and peace. When the tension is removed it is much easier to relax both body and mind. This results in the increased flow of blood to all the tissues, benefiting each and every cell and the lymphatic system resumes its normal function, which is to remove toxins and fight infection in our bodies. Blood pressure, which rises under tension, slowly returns to normal.

When the mind relaxes it becomes calm and peaceful, clarity is restored, muddled thinking vanishes, problems seem easier to solve and new creative ideas arrive out of the blue. As you continue to practise relaxation you will discover the happiness and peace within you. All this has a huge effect on your looks, skin and hair. Nothing is more ageing than tension and nothing is worse for your skin and hair. As you learn to relax mind and body, your skin will regain its radiant glow, your hair regains its bounce and shine due to the circulation being restored in this area, and once you realize that happiness is inside yourself and yours for the taking, the lines of tension will gradually fade away, resulting in a youthful radiance, passion and new energy for living.

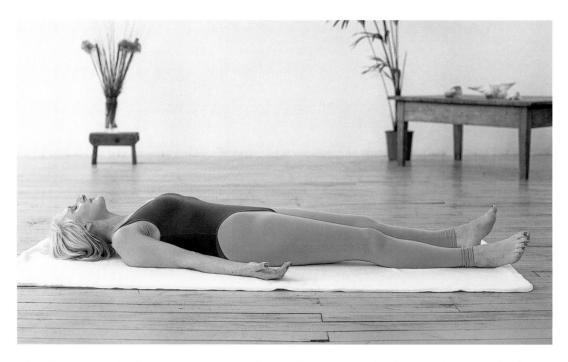

- Lie flat on your back on your mat, your feet about 2 feet apart and your arms, palms uppermost, about 1 foot from your body.
- Make sure that you are warm enough – in colder weather it is wise to cover yourself with a blanket as your temperature may drop as your body relaxes.
- Now slow your breathing down, just breathe calmly, slowly and deeply, inhaling and exhaling through your nose.
- Relax your feet, ankles, and calves.
- Relax your thighs and now feel your legs becoming heavy and really relaxed.
- Relax your abdomen and your back.
- Relax your chest and shoulders.
- Relax your arms and feel them becoming very heavy and just sinking into the floor.
- Smooth out your facial muscles, keeping your breathing slow and deep.

- Let your eyelids become heavy, and roll your eyeballs upwards.
- Let your scalp slide back, and now let your body relax into a calm and dreamy, drowsy state.
- With your body relaxed, visualize beautiful snow-covered mountains sparkling in the sunlight.
- Keep this in your mind and relax, relax, relax.
- Stay there relaxing for 5-10 minutes.
- Slowly dismiss your mountain picture, take a deep breath, stretch your entire body then grab your right knee and gently pull yourself up into a sitting position.

Practise this whenever your feel tired or tense. It works wonders!

15-Minute Miracles
Stage 5

This sequence will dramatically improve the flexibility of both your spine and joints whilst toning, firming and flattening your tummy, strengthening your arms and relieving tightness in your chest. It is great for relieving tension and is very relaxing.

- Three-Limbed Posture
- Pose of a Sage
- Pose of a Boat
- Pose of a Plane
- Wide-Angled Leg Stretch
- Sideways Leg Raise
- Bar of a Gate
- Pose of a Camel
- Pelvic Tilt
- Relaxation

And when you come to a meeting of many ways and do not know which way to choose, do not choose at random, but pause and reflect. Breathe with the trusting deep breaths you took when you first came into the world; let nothing distract you, but wait and go on waiting. Be still and listen in silence to your heart. When it has spoken to you, rise up and follow it.

SUSANNAH TAMARO, FROM *FOLLOW YOUR HEART*

1　Three-Limbed Posture

This is an excellent forwards stretch for the back, releasing tension in the lumbar region. It also helps keep the hips, knees and feet flexible, massages the abdominal organs and is invaluable for promoting their health.

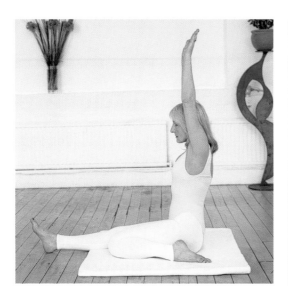
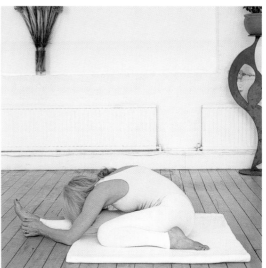

• Sit straight with both legs straight out in front of you. Place your left foot on the left side of your left buttock. Inhale deeply and lift both arms in the air.

• As you exhale, gently bend forwards with your back flat and your head up, to your own maximum position without strain. Your eventual aim is to clasp your right foot and draw your chin to your shin, but your maximum position in the movement will do fine. Hold for a count of 5, increasing to 10 as you progress in the position. Inhale, lift your head and gradually come up into an upright sitting position. Stretch your arms above your head, exhale, relax and repeat on the other side. Repeat the entire sequence once.

Help and Advice
It is really important to notice if one side is more flexible than the other. This can be due to many things, including imbalanced sports and poor posture. However, this movement will really help you correct this potential problem. Sometimes due to stiffness in the knees, ankles and feet, even placing your foot by your buttock can be very difficult in the beginning. Just practise doing just this part of the movement, hold for a count of 5 and then try on the other side. Only when the foot is easily placed by the buttock should you continue with the movement.

2   Pose of a Sage

This movement tones the midriff and waistline, increases the flexibility and tone of the arms while releasing shoulder tension, stretches out the spine and tones the spinal nerves.

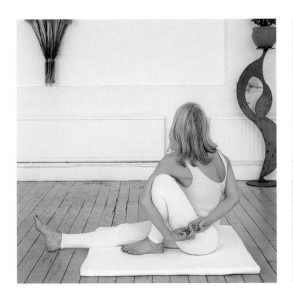
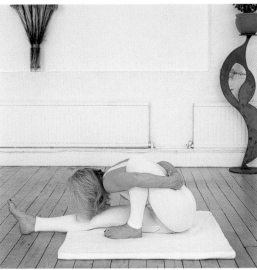

- Sit straight with both legs straight out in front of you. Place your left heel by your left buttock. Place your left arm straight out in front of you on the inside of your left knee and take your right arm back behind your back and aim to join your hands together. (If they can't join, just rest them where they are comfortable.) Now correct your posture and sit very straight, inhale deeply and, as you exhale, rotate your upper body and turn your head over your right shoulder.

- Hold for a count of 5. Inhale and return your body forwards and face over your right leg. Exhale and gently bend forwards into your maximum position without strain. Your eventual aim is to get your chin to your right knee or shin. Hold your maximum forward stretch for a count of 5. Inhale as you return to an upright position. Exhale, relax and repeat to the other side, then repeat the entire sequence once.

Help and Advice
This movement can be very difficult in the beginning – first the hands won't join, second it is difficult to rotate the body keeping your spine straight, and third, even though you can do the Backstretch you may find it difficult to place your chin on your knee in the forward stretch. It is the same for all of us – all I can say is that this movement reaches the bits that all other exercises leave out. Persevere, it will be well worth it! Do remember that you will benefit at every part of this and every other movement.

3   Pose of a Boat

Please do not attempt if you are pregnant

This will strengthen your lower back tone and firm your thighs, strengthen and flatten and firm your tummy whilst helping your concentration and balance.

Caution: If you have a weak back then take great care in the initial phases of this movement.

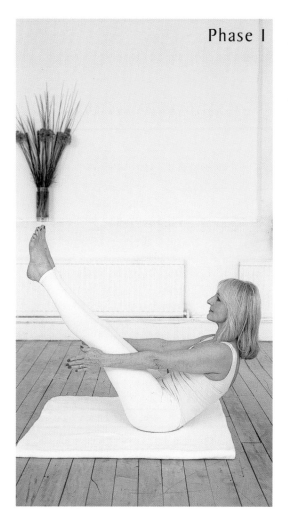

Phase 1

- Sit straight with your legs straight out in front of you on a nice thick mat. Place your arms parallel to your legs.
- Inhale deeply and, as you exhale, gently lean back and lift your legs and balance on your bottom. Hold the position, breathing normally for a count of 1 to start with and building up to 10 as you progress in the movement. Gently lower your legs to the floor, relax and repeat twice.
- Lie flat and draw your knees to your chest and rock your back from side to side to soothe it and relieve lower back tension.

'I had to attend a chiropractor for over 20 years after a rather nasty whiplash accident. Since attending Barbara Currie's yoga classes for some three years, I have not needed any further treatment.'

TERRI, 53

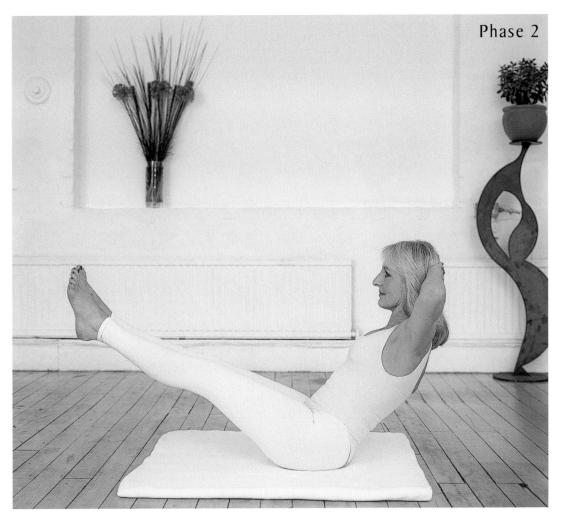

Please only attempt this movement when you are able to do Phase 1 with ease and for a count of 10 three times, as by then your abdominals and back will be stronger.

- Sit straight with both legs stretched out in front of you and interlock your hands behind your head.

- Inhale deeply and, as you exhale, gently lift your legs from the floor. Hold for a count of 1 to start with, increasing to a count of 10 as you progress. Gently lower your legs to the floor and relax. Repeat twice.
- Lie flat on your back, draw your knees to your chest and rock from left to right to soothe your spine.

Help and Advice

Yes, it is strong, but build it up carefully and it will do you the power of good. One frequently finds old people having difficulty getting up from their chairs or supporting their backs as they do, so showing a weakness in the lumbar spine. This clever movement can help tremendously to strengthen the spine and help prevent this problem.

4   Pose of a Plane

This is brilliant for your arms – it gives them great shape and strengthens the wrists, hands and fingers. It also helps to correct posture and releases tension in your lower back.

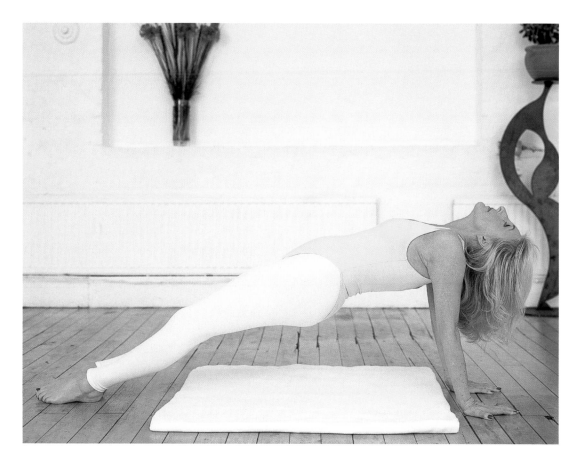

- Sit straight with both legs straight out in front of you. Place your hands comfortably on the floor behind you with your fingertips pointing backwards. They should be about 1 foot behind your bottom.
- Inhale and, as you exhale, lift your body from the floor and balance on your hands and feet.

Ensure that your legs are straight and your body is in a straight line with your head back. Hold for just a count of 1 to start with, increasing this to 10 as you become stronger.
- Lower your bottom slowly to the floor and relax. Repeat once.

Help and Advice
In the beginning it is quite difficult to place your toes on the floor, however this will get easier as you become stronger and lift your body higher.

5   Wide-Angled Leg Stretch

This does wonders for your shape: it really whittles your waist and tones up your midriff and inner thighs, and is good for your back, especially the lumbar region. It is a boon to women, as it can give tremendous help with menstrual problems.

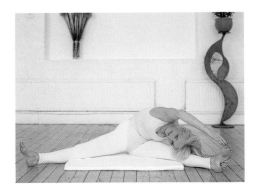

- Sit straight with your legs comfortably wide apart. Inhale and slide your left hand down your left leg towards your left heel as you exhale. Bring your right arm alongside your right ear, with your left hand eventually to your left foot. (This is the aim – remember just to go as far as you can without strain.) Relax in your maximum position for a count of 5. Inhale and slowly return to an upright position, exhale, relax and repeat on the other side.

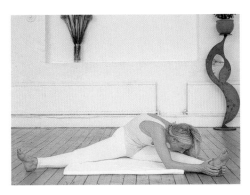

- Now sit with both arms parallel to your left leg, inhale and, as you exhale, bend forwards with your head up and a straight back. Try to clasp your left foot and move as far as you can, eventually aiming your chin to your shin. Relax in your maximum stretch and hold it for a count of 5, then inhale, return to an upright position, exhale and relax. Repeat on the other side.

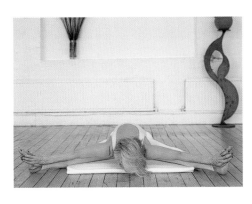

- Finally, sit straight with your legs comfortably wide apart, your arms parallel to your legs, inhale and, as you exhale, carefully stretch forwards keeping your head up and your back straight. Your eventual aim is to have your chin on the floor – this could take many months of practice, but don't worry, you bene-fit tremendously in whatever your maximum posi-tion is for you. Relax and hold for a count of 5, increasing to 10 as you progress. Inhale and return to an upright position. Exhale, relax and repeat twice.

Help and Advice
We have all been there! This position looks impossible – your chin is 3 feet from the floor and your legs won't even open wide. Persevere – please remember we all start like this, and that daily practice and patience are all you need to achieve the maximum stretch. And when you get there it feels great!

6 Sideways Leg Raise

An incredible movement for ensuring the flexibility of the hips and tone of the inner thighs, this is also a great help in relieving lower back tension.

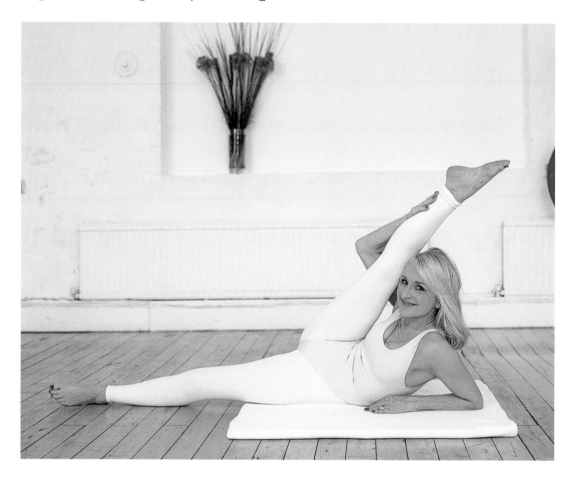

- Lie on your right side with your body in a straight line, one leg on top of the other, and prop yourself up on your right upper arm with your elbow bent and your fingertips pointing to your waist.
- Inhale deeply and, as you exhale, gently lift your left leg and clasp it with your left hand.

Without strain, draw it inwards towards your left ear. Hold your maximum position, breathing normally for a count of 5, then gently lower your leg, relax and repeat. Perform the movement twice on the other side.

Help and Advice
Sometimes when you start this movement your hips can be quite painful. It can help if in the beginning you bend your knee and rotate your hip forwards before carefully lifting it up without strain. With practice the flexibility in your hips will greatly improve.

7   Bar of a Gate

This is excellent for firming and toning your midriff, waistline and inner and outer thighs, and ensuring flexibility in your hips and lower back.

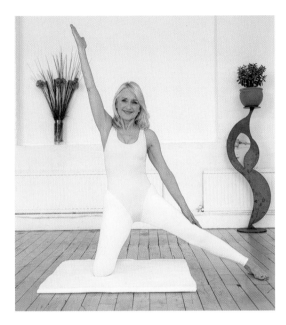
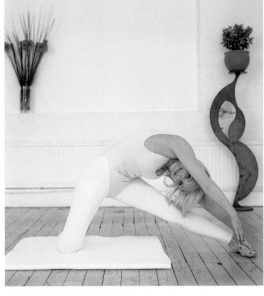

- In a high kneeling position, stretch your left foot out to the left. Place your left hand on your left thigh. Lift your right arm in the air.

- Inhale and, as you exhale, slide your left hand down your left leg and stretch your right arm over as much as possible. Without strain or bending forwards, aim your right hand to touch your left one. Hold your maximum position for a count of 5, increasing to 10 as you progress in the movement. Inhale and slowly return to an upright position. Exhale, relax and repeat. Repeat the entire movement twice to the right.

Help and Advice
It is good to notice if the movement is easier on one side than the other. This is a great movement to help correct lower back and hip imbalances.

8   Pose of a Camel

This is one of my favourites: it opens your chest, releasing tightness, and as a result is a great help for asthmatics. It tones and firms your thighs, firms your jaw and throat, tones your abdominals, gives your spine tremendous flexibility and greatly releases tension.

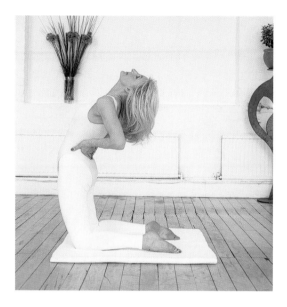
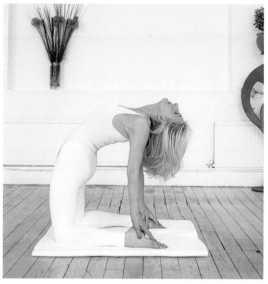

- Adopt a high kneeling position with your knees about 1 foot apart. Place your hands at your waistline with your thumbs in front and your fingers behind. Inhale deeply and, with full lungs, gently relax backwards, keeping your thighs straight and your bottom pushed forwards.

- Arch backwards and drop your hands, aiming the palms of your hands on your feet. (If this is not possible, and it rarely is to start with, just hold your maximum backwards stretch, keeping your hands at your waistline.) Exhale and hold your maximum position for a count of 5, breathing normally. Inhale as you return to an upright position. Exhale and, slowly and carefully, relax forwards, placing your head on the floor in front of your knees, your bottom on your heels and your arms by your sides. Relax in this position, known at the Pose of a Child, for a count of 5, breathing normally. Inhale and slowly return to an upright position. Exhale, relax and repeat.

'I have suffered for many years with sciatica. I started Barbara's yoga classes just over two years ago and have not had any further pain.'

ANNETTE, 64

9 Pelvic Tilt

A lovely movement to tone and tighten your bottom and tummy and release tension in your lower back.

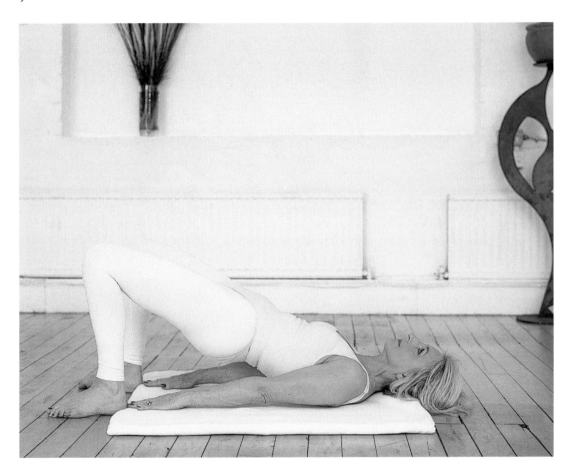

- Lie flat on your back. Place your feet about 1 foot apart and near your bottom. Your fingertips should just touch your heels.
- Inhale deeply and lift your bottom from the floor. In your maximum position, exhale and really tighten your abdomen, pelvic floor and buttocks. Hold this position for a count of 5, breathing normally. Lower your bottom to the floor, relax and repeat 5 times.

- Draw your knees to your chest, interlock your hands around your knees, and gently rock your body from left to right 3 times, then gently let your legs stretch straight out in front of you and relax.

10 Relaxation

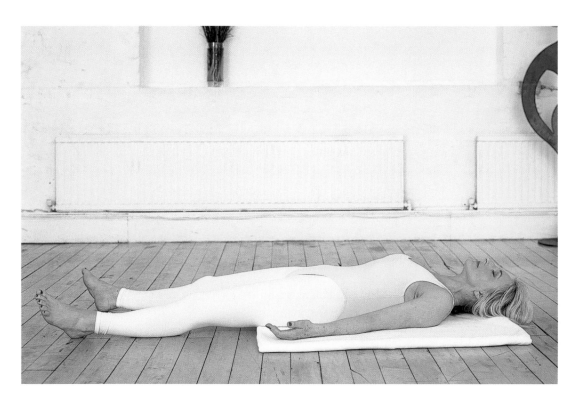

- Lie flat on your back with your arms palms uppermost and 1 foot from your body and your legs 2-3 feet apart. Relax your body as in Stage 4 (page 57). Now close your eyes and visualize a beautiful golden light shining on every cell in your body, warming you, relaxing you and restoring every cell in your body to beautiful, radiant, positive health.

- Keep this in your mind and relax, relax, relax. Stay relaxed for 5–10 minutes, as time permits, then inhale and slowly stretch your body and return to a sitting position.

Well done!

15-Minute Miracles
Stage 6

This sequence includes some of yoga's most wonderful movements. They will firm your throat and jaw, give tremendous flexibility to your spine, slim and tone your midriff and waistline, flatten your tummy, sculpt your thighs to perfection, tone and strengthen your arms, boost your skin and hair and help you relax.

- Pose of a Dog

- Crescent Moon

- Backwards Bend

- Full Twist

- Maltese Cross

- Pose of a Tortoise

- Lowering Your Legs
  to the Floor

- Backstretch

- Sideways Body Raise

- Shoulderstand with
  the Pose of a Fish

- Deep Relaxation

It is not what you do once in a while, it's what you do day in and day out that makes a difference.

JENNY CRAIG

1 Pose of a Dog

It's difficult to adequately express the benefits of this brilliant movement. It increases the flexibility of the spine, stretches the hamstrings and calf muscles and can even help get rid of calciferous spurs on the heels. It strengthens and tones the arms, and relieves tension in the wrists, lower back, neck and shoulders. It is excellent for helping to prevent menstrual cramps and lower backache. It tones the liver, spleen and kidneys and firms the jaw and throat.

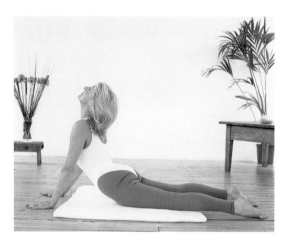

- Lie face-down on your mat and place your hands either side of you in line with your shoulders, your fingertips facing forwards. Place your forehead on the floor. Take a deep breath in. As you exhale, place your chin on the floor. Inhale and, keeping your lower abdomen on the floor, slowly lift your upper body from the floor into the Pose of a Cobra. Stretch into the movement as far as you can without strain, drop your head back and relax in your maximum position. Exhale and hold for a count of 5, breathing normally.

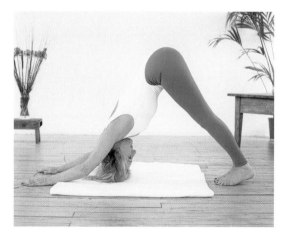

- Inhale deeply and, as you exhale, tuck your toes under and, pushing down hard on your hands, lift your bottom in the air and aim to stretch your heels to the floor, drawing your head down between your arms so that your body resembles an inverted 'V'. Hold this position for a count of 5, then slowly swing your head back up between your arms, bend your elbows and gently lower your body to the floor. Relax and repeat once to start with, but as your strength, ability and agility improve increase to 3 repeats. Well done!

Help and Advice
At first it can be quite difficult to move into the inverted 'V' position. If this is a problem for you, then gently move onto your knees first and then take your heels to the floor.

2   Crescent Moon

This is a lovely backwards bend. It firms your thighs and jaw, releases tension in your chest, stimulates your kidneys and adrenal glands and gives your spine tremendous flexibility.

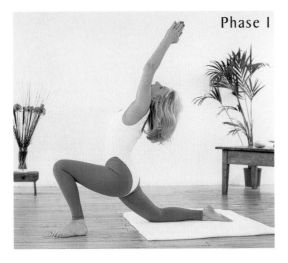

Phase 1

- Kneel on a thick mat. Place your left foot flat on the floor about 3 feet in front of your right knee but in line with your left knee. Place both hands on your left knee.
- Inhale deeply and push your left buttock forwards, aiming your left buttock towards your left heel, so stretching out your right leg. The front of the right calf should now be flat on the floor.
- Lift both your arms up in the air, placing your palms together and crossing your thumbs. Drop your head back and look at your crossed thumbs. Hold your maximum position in this movement, breathing normally for a count of 5. Lower your arms, relax and repeat to the other side.

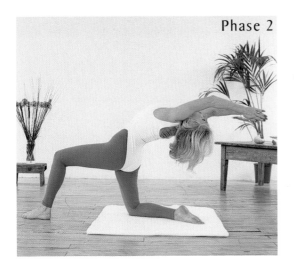

Phase 2

Please don't even attempt to move on to this phase until you can do Phase 1 with ease.

- In the maximum position in Phase 1, concentrate on your thumbs, take a deep breath and slowly and carefully aim to bend backwards, exhaling in your maximum position. Hold for a count of 5, breathing normally. Inhale as you return to an upright position, exhale, relax and repeat on the other side. Repeat the entire sequence.

Help and Advice
Starting to bend backwards in this movement is difficult at first. Don't worry, even an inch is progress – and again, with daily practice, it just gets better and better.

3   Backwards Bend

This delightful pose relieves tightness and tension in the chest, firms the neck and throat, corrects poor posture, strengthens the wrists, tones the upper arms and is a fantastic firmer for the thighs.

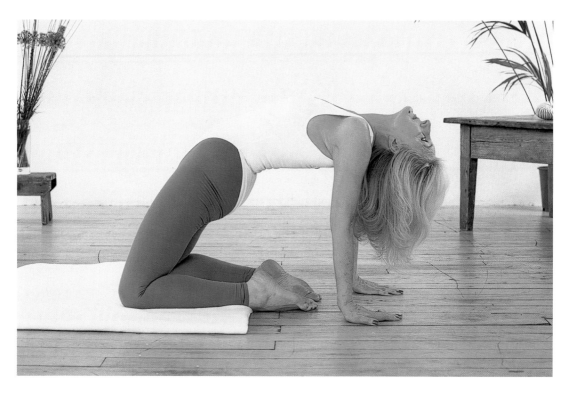

- Kneel on a thick mat and place your hands flat on the floor behind you.
- Take a deep breath in and gently lift your bottom from your heels. Exhale in your maximum position and, breathing normally, hold for a count of 5, increasing to 10 as you progress in the position.

- Gently lower your bottom to your heels, relax and carefully take your head to the floor in front of your knees, placing your hands by your sides. This is the Pose of a Child. Stay in this position for a count of 5, breathing normally, then inhale and return to a kneeling position. Repeat twice.

Help and Advice
Due to stiffness in the knee joints, a lot of people find this movement quite difficult and that sitting on their heels is uncomfortable. This can be helped by placing a blanket folded up between your bottom and heels and then performing the movement by placing your hands on the floor but not lifting your bottom until your knees feel a bit better.

If your knees are very stiff, just practise kneeling every day without doing the movement. Very soon they will become more flexible.

4 Full Twist

Only attempt this movement when you can do the Simple Twist in Stage 4 with ease. The Full Twist is wonderful for releasing tension and improving flexibility in the entire spine. It stimulates extra blood flow to the spinal nerves. It increases flexibility in the lower back, hips and shoulders, slims the midriff, waistline and hips, and firms the neck, jaw and throat.

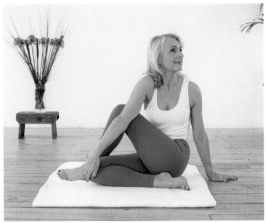

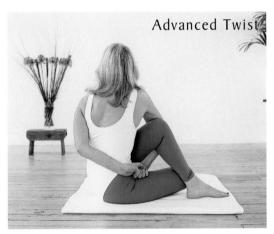

Advanced Twist

- Sit straight with both legs straight out in front of you. Place your right foot between your legs, with your right heel by your groin.
- Inhale and bring your left foot over your right thigh, placing your left heel on the floor on the outer side of your right thigh. Exhale and place your left hand on the floor behind your back.
- Take a deep breath and, as you exhale, take your right arm over your left knee and place it on your right knee. Inhale deeply and, as you exhale, carefully rotate your body and turn your head over your left shoulder. Hold this position for a count of 5, breathing normally, increasing to 10 as you progress in the movement. Slowly inhale and return your body to face the front, exhale, relax and repeat on the other side. Then repeat the entire movement.

- For a stronger stretch, in the maximum movement slide your right hand under your left thigh, take your left hand behind your back and try to join them together. Hold this position for a count of 5, then relax and repeat on the other side.

Help and Advice
Initial attempts at this movement can have a very humbling effect, as it really reveals the stiffness in our joints. Don't despair, even if you feel that your co-ordination and flexibility are non-existent in the beginning, with practice your youthful flexibility will return.

5 Maltese Cross

I love this sequence, it is a woman's dream: it tones and flattens the tummy whilst firming all the muscles in the legs, sculpting and streamlining the upper thighs and releasing lower back tension. It keeps the hips beautifully flexible and can help people with painful hips and sciatica.

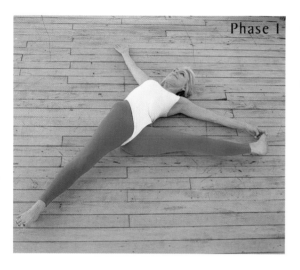

Phase 1

- Lie flat on your back. Place both feet together and spread your arms open wide so that you resemble a cross.
- Take a deep breath in and, as you exhale, keeping your left heel on the floor gently stretch your left foot up to your left hand. Your eventual aim is to be able to grab your left big toe in your left hand, but don't worry, your maximum position will do fine. Hold for a count of 5, then slowly draw your foot back to its starting position. Repeat on the other side, then repeat twice on each side.

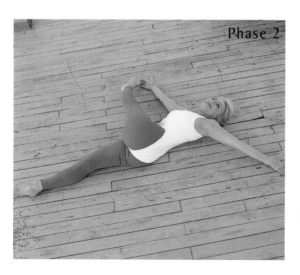

Phase 2

- Lie flat on your mat with both feet together and your arms outstretched at shoulder level, palms uppermost.
- Take a deep breath in and lift your left leg in the air, aiming to place your left foot in the centre of your right hand. Again, remember not to strain – your maximum position, whatever it may be, is just fine. Hold your maximum position for a count of 5, breathing normally.
- Inhale and lift your left leg carefully, pointing your toes to the ceiling. Then, keeping it straight, slowly lower it. Repeat on the other side, then repeat twice on each side.

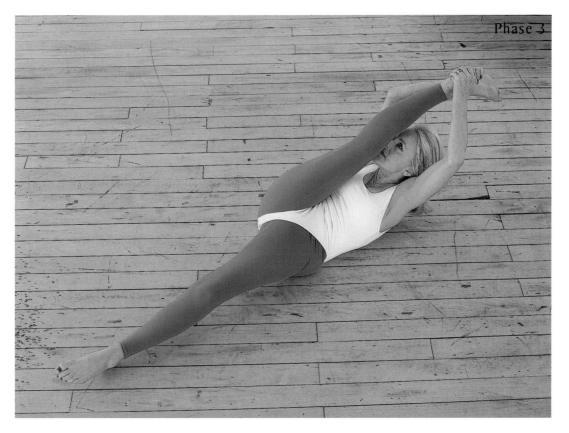

- Lie flat on your back on your mat and place your arms palms uppermost flat on the floor behind your head. Place your legs together.
- Inhale. Lift your right leg in the air, keeping it straight. Clasp it wherever you can reach it and draw your right knee towards your right nostril. Your eventual aim is to be able to clasp your big toe and aim your right knee to your right nostril. This can, however, take many months of practice; as always, your best movement without strain will do fine.

- Hold your maximum movement, breathing normally, for a count of 5. Exhale slowly, lower your leg, take your arms slowly back to behind your head and relax. Repeat on the other side, then repeat the entire sequence twice.

Help and Advice
The biggest temptation in both Phase 1 and 2 is to roll over a little onto your side to make the movement easier. Please don't, keep your shoulders and hips in their correct position and your eyes fixed on the ceiling. Even if your progress is slower you will benefit much more from this wonderful sequence.

6 Pose of a Tortoise

This is an excellent movement for relieving stiffness in the lower back and hips. It tones the abdominal organs and the spine. It is a very soothing and refreshing movement, giving you a lovely feeling of relaxed calm after a relatively long stay in the movement.

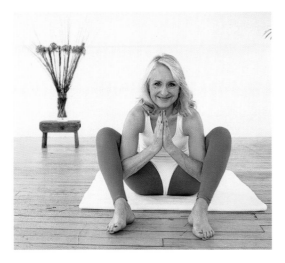

- Sit with your legs about 1 foot apart and your feet flat on the floor. Place your hands in prayer. Inhale and lower your elbows towards the floor.

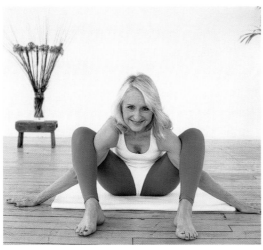

- As you exhale, gently open your elbows and stretch your hands under your knees, placing them on the floor on the outer side of your knees. Now in your maximum stretch, notice the position of your elbows. If they are on the outer side of your knees, you will be able to continue the movement. If not, just relax in your maximum position and hold for 5, breathing normally.

'Taking up yoga two years ago at 68 may well be thought to be a classic case of closing the stable door – albeit the old horse more limped than bolted away! Not so. I had joined the booming "bad back club" when the physio recommended continuing treatment through yoga – but she didn't tell me about the two big bonuses. Even as a disgrace to yoga, I am not just a bit but a very worthwhile bit more flexible, and I really feel so much fitter overall – dare I say, younger even. I find the "whole body" approach convincing. And the second big bonus? Barbara's informed and inspirational teaching. I'll eat my yoga blanket if it doesn't come through in her writing.'

DAVID, 70

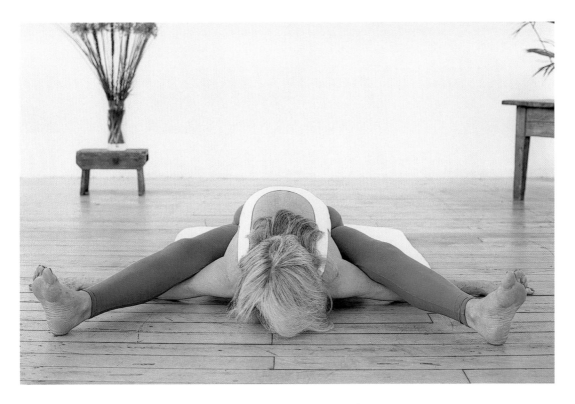

- To continue the movement, take another breath then stretch your legs out as wide as possible. As you stretch forwards, stretch your arms out as wide as possible. Relax in your maximum position without strain, aiming your chin to the floor, and hold for a count of 10, breathing normally. Inhale and, slowly and carefully, draw your feet in first, then your arms, and inhale as you return to the starting position. Exhale, relax and repeat once. Only when you can achieve the maximum stretch in the Tortoise with your chin on the floor and your arms and legs at full stretch, you might like to try the advanced Tortoise.

Advanced Tortoise

- For this, in your maximum Tortoise stretch, gently take your arms behind your back and try to join your hands. Hold for 5, relax, unclasp your hands, draw your feet in first and return slowly to your upright position. Relax.
- Repeat once.

Help and Advice
No, it's not easy. Just practise at your own pace and you will be rewarded handsomely.

7   Lowering Your Legs to the Floor

Caution: If you have a weak lower back, please read 'Help and Advice' first.

This movement is one of the best for helping you to that beautiful flat, toned yoga tummy.

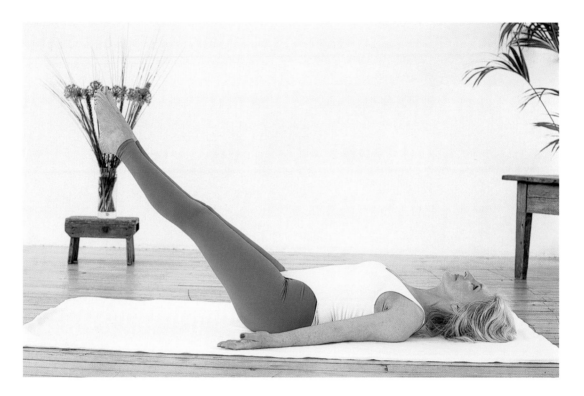

- Lie flat on your back with your arms by your sides.
- Bend your knees and gently lift your legs until they are at right angles to the floor.
- Inhale deeply and, as you exhale, carefully lower your legs all the way to the floor, keep-ing them straight. (In the beginning it is best to lower your legs fairly quickly, only slowing the movement down as your muscles become stronger.) Relax and repeat 3 times, increasing to 6 times as you progress in the movement.

Help and Advice

When you do this to begin with you may find that this movement is too strong for your lower back. If this is the case, then lower your legs a little and when you feel the tiniest suggestion of a pull in the lower back, bend your knees and continue to lower your legs to the floor keeping your knees bent. Continue to practise like this and you will find that gradually you are able to lower your legs a little bit more until eventually you are able to lower them all the way to the floor without needing to bend them. You will then have con-siderably strengthened your lower back muscles and your abdominals.

8   Backstretch

We first tried this yoga essential in Stage 4, page 49. Now let's see what wonderful progress you have made!

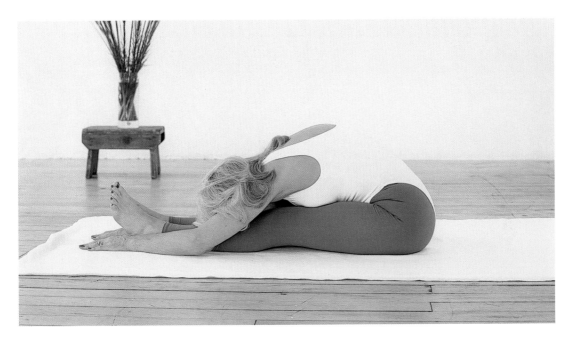

- Sit straight up on your mat. Inhale and lift both your arms up in the air.
- Exhale and, slowly and carefully, move forwards with a straight back, head up in your own maximum position without strain. Your eventual aim is to clasp your heels and draw your chin to your shins. Remember, your maximum position, wherever it may be, is fine.

- Hold your maximum stretch, relaxing in it and breathing normally for a count of 10. Inhale and lift your head. Slowly return to an upright position. Exhale, relax and repeat twice.

'It was my doctor who recommended that I start yoga classes. I'd been diagnosed with Irritable Bowel Syndrome and he thought that yoga would help. It's been great – not only has my IBS cleared up, but I'm more relaxed, I can deal with stress much better and I'm more toned. It's made such a difference in the year and a half I've been practising that I'll definitely keep it up.'

LISA, 24

9 Sideways Body Raise

This is an amazing toner and strengthener for the arms, giving them a fabulous shape. It is a weight-bearing movement and so can help to prevent osteoporosis; it is a balance movement and so helps your powers of concentration. It is excellent for the wrist, stretching it out, and can help to prevent carpal tunnel syndrome.

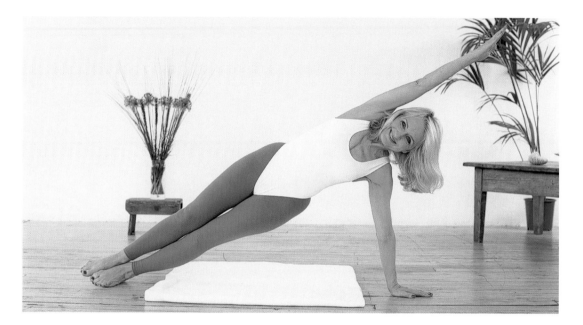

- Sit on the floor with your hands about 1 foot apart to the right of your body. Keep your knees bent and ensure that your hands and feet are on a non-slip surface. (If you have previously had a shoulder or wrist injury, then transfer a little of your weight to your hands in this position, but do not lift your body from the floor until you have regained your strength.) Inhale and, as you exhale, lift your body from the floor and ensure that both hands and both feet support your weight.

- Now adjust your body so that your right shoulder is directly above your right wrist and your arm is straight. Lift your bottom and ensure that your left foot is on top of your right one and that your body is in a straight line.
- When and only when you feel strong enough, lift your left arm from the floor and stretch it in a straight line with your left ear. Focus on a spot on the floor to help your balance and hold for a count of 5. Lower your bottom to the floor, relax and repeat on the other side. Repeat the whole sequence once more.

Help and Advice
Our automatic response is to put a hand out to break a fall should we slip; this can frequently result in a fracture if we have weak wrists and arms. This movement addresses this problem perfectly. If you have had an arm problem, then just put a little weight on your hands at first and gradually build up your strength until you are able to do the full movement.

10 Shoulderstand with the Pose of a Fish

This movement is called 'the mother of yoga postures' and is the second most important yoga exercise – the first being the Headstand. It has wonderful benefits: it stimulates excellent blood flow to the skin and hair, and has a very rejuvenating effect on them. It also helps to reverse the adverse ageing effects of gravity.

By stimulating extra blood flow to the thyroid and parathyroid glands in the neck, it helps keep them in good condition and can revitalize a sluggish metabolism.

It is excellent for the health of the legs and can help prevent varicose veins, haemorrhoids and thread veins. It strengthens the spine, legs and abdominal muscles, and the extra blood flow to the chest can be beneficial for asthma sufferers. The extra blood flow to the brain can help headache sufferers, benefit the brain itself and improve eyesight and hearing.

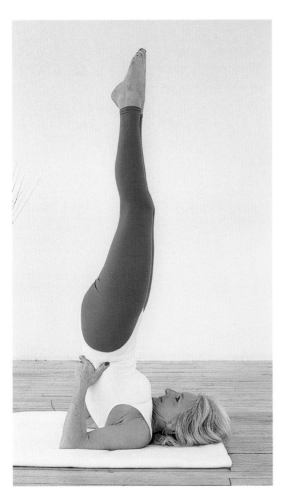

- Lie flat on your back with your hands by your side. Take a deep breath in and, as you exhale, gently bend your knees and lift your lower body from the floor. Support your back by placing your hands at your waistline. Continue to lift your legs until your body is in a perfect straight line. This may take a while to achieve – do your best and then relax in your maximum movement. Hold your maximum position in this movement for a count of 10 to start with, increasing at the rate of about 30 seconds per week until, with practice, you are holding for about 3 minutes. To come out of the posture, draw your knees to your forehead and then gently roll down your back about one vertebra at a time until your bottom touches the floor.

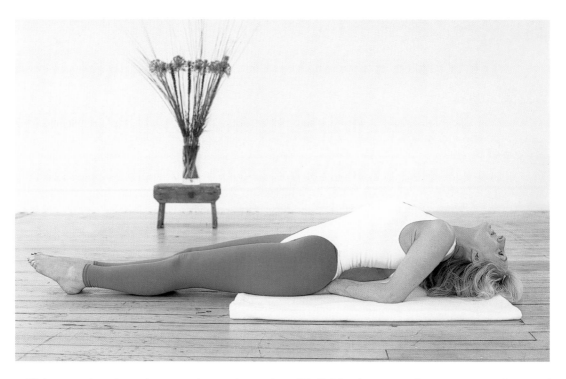

- Slide your hands under your buttocks and bring the top of your head onto the floor. Relax in this position, which is called the Pose of a Fish. Take a deep breath, hold for a count of 5, then exhale slowly and lower your upper body to the floor. Lie flat, close your eyes and relax.

To finish, draw your knees to your chest and rock very gently from left to right to soothe your back and let it relax into the floor. Let both legs go straight out in front of you. Close your eyes and relax. Do not repeat.

Help and Advice

If you can't manage the Shoulderstand, you can obtain similar benefits for your legs by lying flat on your back and keeping your upper body and bottom on the floor, placing your feet on a wall or on a chair to elevate them. This is lovely and really relaxing, good for tired legs, and can help varicose veins.

11 Deep Relaxation

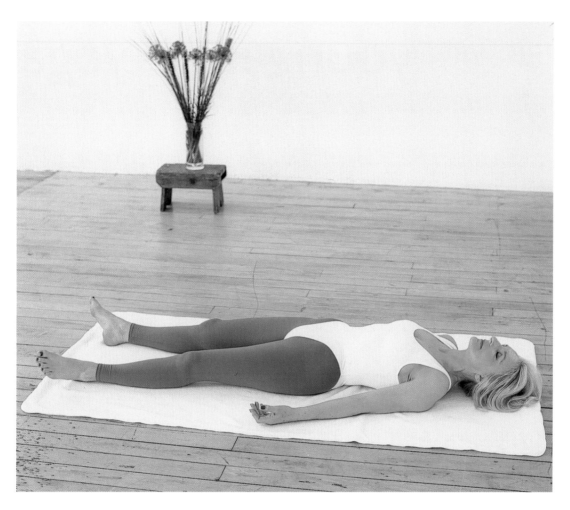

- Lie flat on your mat, slow your breathing down and relax each area of your body in turn as we did in Stage 4.
- Now imagine that you are lying on a beautiful beach with lovely blue waves lapping on the shore.

- You are peaceful, relaxed and calm. Warm sunlight is bathing your body and the waves are lulling you into a dreamy and drowsy state. Now, as you inhale slowly, visualize the waves drifting towards you and, as you exhale, visualize them slowly drifting back out to sea again. Do this with every breath and relax, relax, relax.

Part Two

growing **younger** with **yoga**

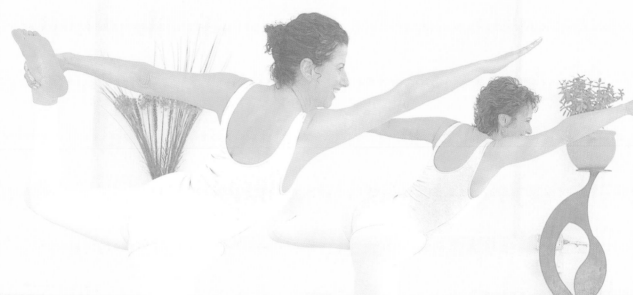

In this book I have so far aimed to give you an excellent grounding in the major yoga movements. Practising these every day will keep your spine and joints flexible, tone 100 per cent of your body both inside and out, stretch away your tensions, give you energy, improve your breathing and help you relax and sleep well, while at the same time dramatically improving your shape and boosting the condition of your skin and hair.

Most of us, however, have specific areas of mind or body that we would like to improve, and so in the chapters that follow I will show you my favourite movements to help with these specific body challenges. Then we'll end with yoga's amazing advanced movements and brilliant rejuvenating inverted postures. All you need to do is choose a sequence and incorporate it into your daily 15-minute session, doing it either as well as or instead of your a.m. (Stages 1–3) or p.m. (Stages 4–6) stretch.

Note: Please do not replace your 15-minute a.m. or p.m. stretches with these movements entirely. Instead, do them on alternate days.

Remember to work slowly and carefully – and never, ever strain yourself.

Your 15-Minute Facial

This sequence will tone and firm your face and jawline, bringing back youthful contours. It will smooth away tension from your brow, boost the condition of your skin and hair, help revitalize your eyesight, release stress, help you to instant calm and deep relaxation and take 15 years off the way you look and feel.

- Jaw Exercises

- Forehead Smoother

- The Lion Exercise

- Scalp Exercise

- Eye Exercises

- Head and Neck Exercises

- Alternate Nostril Breathing Exercise

- Pose of a Plough

- Deep Relaxation

Just trust yourself, then you will know how to live.

GOETHE

1 Jaw Exercises

Yoga is excellent for the tone and firmness of the jaw and throat. The Backwards Bends and Twists are ideal for this.

However, there are times when we need to speed things up a bit, so here are my two favourites. They do absolute wonders for firming the jaw and getting rid of a double chin.

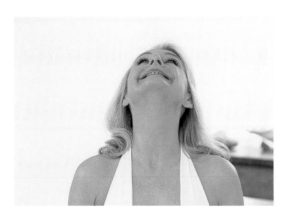

Jaw Exercise 1

- Sit with your back straight and grin from ear to ear.
- While grinning, let your head carefully drop backwards and, keeping it there, still grinning, open and close your mouth very slowly 3 times.
- Slowly return to an upright position, relax and repeat twice.

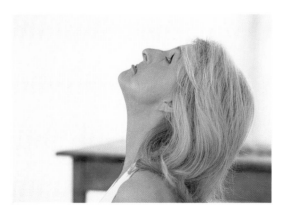

Jaw Exercise 2

- Some people don't get a double chin but instead experience sagging in the middle portion of the neck – the so-called 'turkey neck'. This movement is an excellent aid to correcting this and giving you a beautiful, firm, swanlike neck.
- Sit straight and gently drop your head back.
- With your head dropped back, gently take your bottom set of teeth up towards your nose (you won't make the connection, so don't worry). Hold this position for a count of 5, then relax and repeat 3 times.

2 Forehead Smoother

This is genius, it is almost unbelievably soothing and really helps smooth out those tense and ageing tramlines.

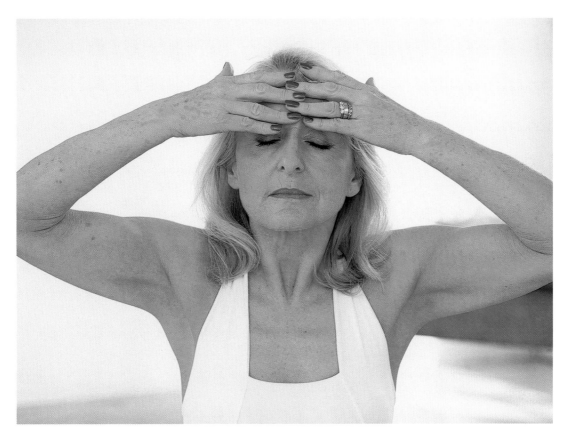

- Sit straight and close your eyes. Now gently endeavour to smooth your brow by taking your scalp back and dropping your eyebrows.
- Place your fingertips, interleaved, in the centre of your forehead.
- Inhale deeply and, as you exhale very slowly, whilst counting to 7, slide your fingers over your brow to your hairline. Relax and repeat at least 5 times, aiming eventually to do 10. Now look at yourself in the mirror. The results are immediately visible. Do this whenever tension strikes. It is also excellent to help prevent the onset of a headache; if you are able to cool your fingers first, the results are even more stress-relieving and soothing.

3 The Lion Exercise

This movement stimulates blood flow to your face, so invigorating the skin. It tones the muscles of the face and neck, giving you an excellent 'face-lift'. It stimulates blood flow to the back of the throat and is a wonderful aid in helping to relieve a sore throat. By opening the eyes very wide, it tones the eye muscles and the delicate skin surrounding the eyes. This movement has excellent benefits – but do it alone because it looks dreadful!

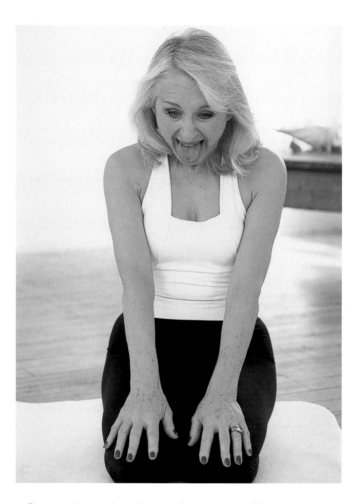

- Sit straight in a kneeling or classic crossed-leg position and place your hands on your knees.
- Inhale deeply, then exhale forcibly and simultaneously stick your tongue out, aiming it to curl over your chin, stretch your hands out wide and open your eyes as wide as possible. Hold for a count of 10, then inhale, relax and repeat 3 times.

4   Scalp Exercise

Have you noticed how your hair reflects your state of mind? Tension literally strangles our tissues and can inhibit blood flow to our hair follicles – this can leave our hair looking limp and tired.

This simple massage releases this tension and is excellent for stimulating healthy blood flow to the hair roots, so improving the condition of the hair dramatically. It is best done before you shampoo your hair or at night before you sleep. It is, however, very relaxing and invigorating to the scalp at any time.

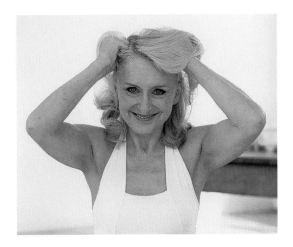

- Sit in a comfortable position and spread out your fingers in your hair so that they are lying on your scalp. Clasp your hair, now slightly pull it and move the scalp by gently pulling and making 3 circles with the hair. Transfer your hands to another area and repeat. Keep doing this until the entire scalp has been thoroughly massaged. The whole scalp should tingle and feel alive and refreshed.

'I do lots of general exercise, but my two main interests are running and yoga. I first got into yoga because I thought the stretching exercises would really complement my running, and a friend recommended Barbara's classes to me. I've been practising for two and a half years now and, as well as the stretches helping with my running, yoga has toned and strengthened me. It's something that I'll definitely be sticking with.'

LIZ, 26

5 Eye Exercises

The eyes need exercises to keep them in good condition, to strengthen the muscles, stimulate blood flow to the optic nerve and help prevent the lens stiffening. These movements do just that and can really help your eyesight. I find that a lot of my students, after practising these movements, tell me that they are delighted to report that they no longer need their reading glasses!

These exercises are particularly beneficial if, like a lot of people these days, you spend hour after hour on a computer.

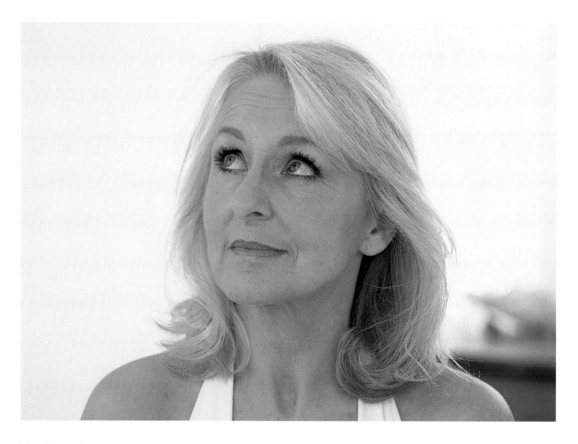

Eye Exercise 1

- Sit straight and imagine an enormous clock in front of you. Look upward to a maximum upwards stretch towards 12 o'clock. Hold for a count of 3 in this position, now move your eyes to 1 o'clock, and again hold for a count of 3. Continue in this way round the clock until you once again arrive at 12 o'clock. Now go back the other way, moving your eyes to 11 o'clock and holding for 3, etc. Continue round the clock until you once more reach 12 o'clock.

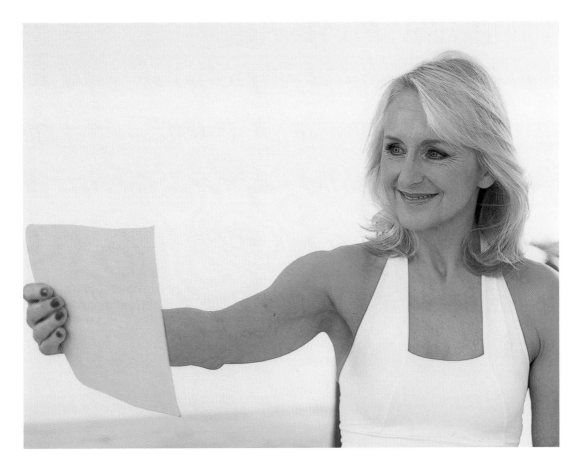

Eye Exercise 2

- Find two pieces of print, one quite large that you are able to read easily without glasses or contact lenses, and one that you have difficulty in reading but can just about manage in good light. Paste these pieces of print into a notebook.

- Look at them at least three times a day in excellent light 1) at comfortable reading distance; 2) with your arm stretched out as far as possible; and 3) as near to your face as you can bring it before it goes blurry. Do this every day and you will find your eyesight benefiting. When this becomes easy for you, then try two smaller pieces of print and continue. Once you have regained confidence in your ability to strengthen your eyesight, use this exercise with pieces of small print in your daily life i.e. ingredients on bottles, etc., and continue to make it a lifetime habit. (On a personal note, I am most grateful to have been taught these movements, as now at 60 years of age I have no need for glasses. I love being able to see clearly, and find it very easy to fit these movements into the busiest day.)

- After doing your eye exercises, rub the palms of your hands together to warm them, then place your warmed hands over your closed eyes and stay in this position, breathing calmly and slowly for a count of 30. Then lower your hands, slowly open your eyes and relax. This is known as 'palming' the eyes, and is most refreshing for tired or strained eyes.

6 Head and Neck Exercises

These movements firm and tone the jaw and neck and release tension in the neck that causes headaches and restricts blood flow to the brain. They can remove osteophytes or tiny calcium deposits that so often settle in the neck and cause stiffness. They are most beneficial for headache sufferers.

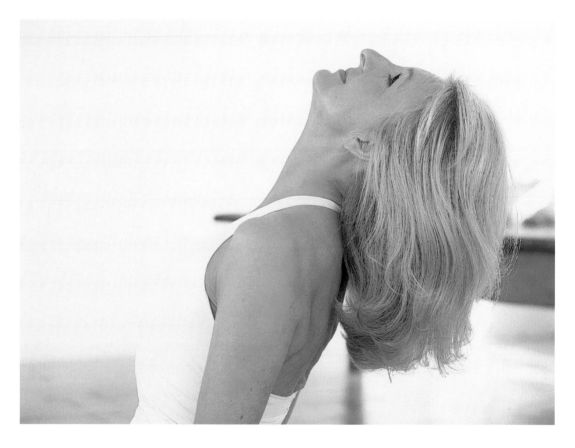

- Sit in either a crossed-leg or kneeling position and make sure that your spine is straight. Do not strain. (Note: if you have a very tense or tight neck, then only move a minuscule amount to begin with, making a tiny circle and progressing carefully as you improve.)

- Close your eyes and drop your head gently forwards, then carefully roll your head to the right, gently and slowly roll it backwards, roll it to the left and then slowly forwards. Make 3 slow careful circles to the right and follow with 3 to the left. This is blissfully relaxing – enjoy it.

7 Alternate Nostril Breathing Exercise

This soothing and calming movement relieves tension that plays havoc with your skin, hair and energy flow. It is really calming. Remember that how you are on the outside is a reflection of what is going on inside, so use this whenever tension strikes.

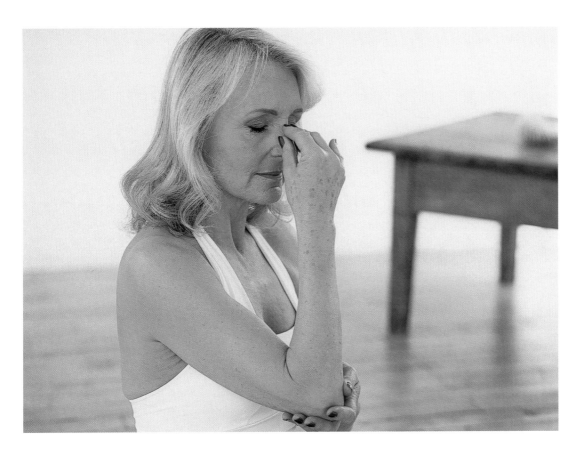

- Sit comfortably in either a crossed-leg or kneeling position or, if more convenient, in a comfortable chair. Close your eyes.
- Place your right thumb on your right nostril, your next two fingers on the bridge of your nose and your next finger on your left nostril. Support your right elbow with your left hand. Unblock your right nostril and, keeping your left one blocked, inhale for a count of 5.

- Block the right nostril and, keeping both nostrils closed, hold the breath for a count of 5. Unblock your left nostril and slowly exhale for a count of 5. Inhale through your left nostril for a count of 5. Hold for 5 and exhale through the right nostril for 5.

Continue this slow, beautiful relaxing breathing exercise for 10 rounds. It will help you relax and cope with even the most upsetting situation, and is excellent to do before going to sleep.

8   Pose of a Plough

Now you have firmed your jaw and facial muscles, soothed your brow, worked your eye muscles and released the stresses and strains within you, it is a wonderful thing to relax into the Pose of a Plough. This posture will stimulate blood flow to your face, scalp, brain and eyes and release tension in your lower back.

If you do have the above problems, then lie down and relax and we will join you in a minute.

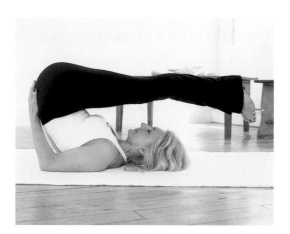

- Lie down flat on your mat on your back. Inhale and bend your knees, and slowly and carefully lift your bottom from the floor. Place your hands on your lower back to support it, and aim to have your legs parallel to the floor in the first instance.

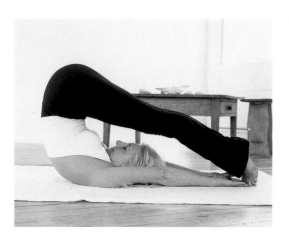

- Relax in your maximum position without strain and hold for a count of 10 to start, increasing to a count of 30 as you progress in the movement. Your eventual aim is to have your toes on the floor and your fingertips stretched back to touch your toes. Gently lower your knees to your forehead and slowly roll down your back one vertebra at a time until your bottom reaches the floor, then stretch both legs straight out in front of you, lie flat and relax. Draw both knees to your chest, interlock your hands around them and gently rock from side to side, then stretch both legs straight out in front of you and relax.

'Since starting yoga classes five years ago, I feel younger slimmer, more agile and more in tune with my body. Every morning I do 15-20 minutes of yoga which leaves me invigorated and energized and ready to start the day! I couldn't do without it now!'

CAROL, 54

9 Deep Relaxation

Lie flat on your back with your legs about 2 feet apart and your arms 1 foot from your body. Make sure that you are warm enough. Slow your breathing down and relax each muscle in turn.

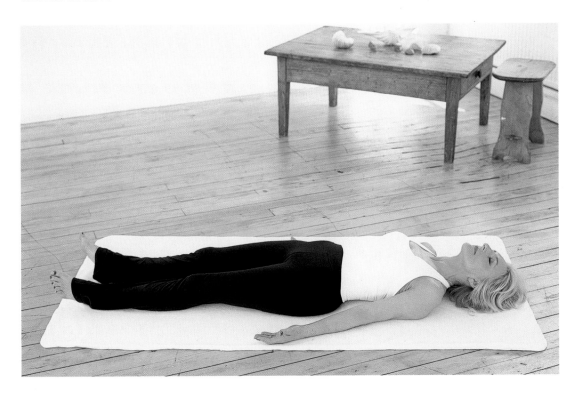

- Now visualize a very beautiful red rose. Concentrate on the rich velvety colour of the petals, keep this in your mind and relax, relax, relax.
- Stay relaxed for 5 to 10 minutes, depending on your schedule, and then gently stretch your body from top to toe.

- Grasp your right knee in both hands, inhale deeply and pull yourself gently into a sitting position.

Skin Care

The movements you have just performed, together with the inverted postures that begin on page 135, are, in my opinion, the best, most natural and rejuvenating facelift possible. I believe you have to take care of your skin, but I don't believe that this need cost a fortune. Over the years I, perhaps like you, have been tempted from time to time by some of the many expensive 'miracle' creams on the market. I have to admit I have never noticed any difference in my skin. Nowadays my personal routine is simple, inexpensive and uncomplicated. I use a L'Oreal cleanser and skin tonic from their 'Plenitude' range, followed by a little Estee Lauder 'Eye Zone' gel around my eyes. On my skin I use Estee Lauder's 'Night Repair' followed by her 'Resilience' day and night cream. After my shower I massage my entire body in one of a variety of body moisturizers. I do not have facials or any other beauty treatment apart from a 3-monthly haircut and highlights, manicure and pedicure session.

If due to unforeseen circumstances I am not able to get out in the fresh air, exercise, eat the foods I enjoy or drink enough water, I see the detrimental effects on my skin and facial contours immediately. I was very pleased to hear that two of the best beauty editors in this country, having done an in-depth analysis of skin care products in their brilliant, most beautiful and informative book *The 21st Century Beauty Bible*, Sarah Stacey and Josephine Fairley state that good things for the skin are:

- deep rhythmic breathing
- water – try to drink 2 litres per day
- fresh fruit and vegetables
- good fats, as found in oily fish – mackerel, pilchards, sardines, salmon, tuna, herrings and trout
- good sleep
- laughter, happiness and peace of mind.

I totally agree with all the above, and with the quote that ends their book, which is from Audrey Hepburn:

True beauty in a woman is reflected in her soul. It is the caring that she lovingly gives and the passion that she shows. And the beauty of a woman with passing years only grows.

So, cleanse, tone and nourish your skin with your favourite products, but also stretch into your yoga postures to stimulate extra blood flow to your skin and hair, breathe deeply, sleep well, eat well and live, love, laugh and enjoy every moment of your life. This is the best beauty treatment in the world.

Arms, Neck and Shoulders

These movements are excellent for relieving tension in the neck and shoulders, correcting poor posture, firming the muscles that support the bust and firming and toning the upper arms. They will strengthen the arms, elbow and wrists, keep your joints flexible, help your balance and concentration and help you relax and stay calm. Movements 6–11 are arm balances; their main benefits are to strengthen the arms, elbows and wrists, help to prevent osteoporosis and give that beautiful firm, lean yoga shape.

Movements 8–11 are not easy movements, so go carefully. Select only 1 in the initial stages and do it no more than twice until you are able and strong enough to perform it with ease. Continue until you are able to perform all four movements and then (only when you feel strong enough) do more than 1 movement each time you practise yoga.

- Pose of a Mountain
- Pose of a Cow
- Chest Expansion
- Head of a Horse
- Finger Exercises
- Sideways Body Raise
- Pose of a Plane
- Pose of a Crow
- Pose of Eight Curves
- Pose of an Elephant
- Pose of a Firefly
- Relaxation

If we think of defeat that is what we get, if we are undecided nothing will happen for us, we must pick something great to do and do it. Never think of failure at all, for as we think that is what we will get.

MAHARISHI MAHESH YOGI

1 Pose of a Mountain

This movement is excellent for releasing neck and shoulder tension, firming and toning the upper arms and is invaluable for correcting posture.

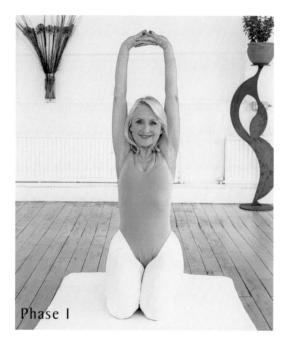

Phase 1

- Kneel down with your bottom on your heels (if this is difficult, place a cushion between your bottom and heels).
- Interlock your hands in front of you; now turn them 'inside-out' so that you are looking at the backs of your hands. Inhale and lift your arms up above your head, ensuring that the 'inside' of your arms are in line with your ears, your back is straight and your hands are directly above your head.
- Hold this position for a count of 5, breathing normally. Then exhale, lower your arms and relax. Repeat 3 times.

    When, and only when, you can sit on your heels with ease, then you may try this more advanced stage of the movement.

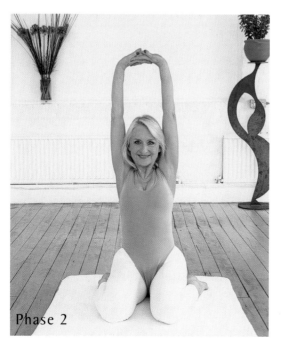

Phase 2

- In a high kneeling position, open your knees hip-width apart. Place your hands on your heels and, carefully and without strain, aim to lower your bottom to the floor between your heels.
- When the above kneeling position is possible, interlock your hands in front of you and lift your arms in the air as in the previous position.
- Hold for a count of 5, breathing normally, then undo your arms, relax and repeat 3 times.

Extra Benefits from Phase 2

This is so good for keeping your knees and hips flexible, and is excellent for correcting poor posture and straightening your back.

100

2 Pose of a Cow

This movement, although humbling at first as it can show how stiff and imbalanced our shoulders have become, is fantastic. We were first introduced to this movement in Stage 1. Now let's see how you have progressed. The movement is invaluable for rebalancing the shoulders, releasing shoulder tension, correcting posture and firming and toning your upper arms. Phase 2 is excellent for aiding the flexibility and tone of your hips, knees and ankles.

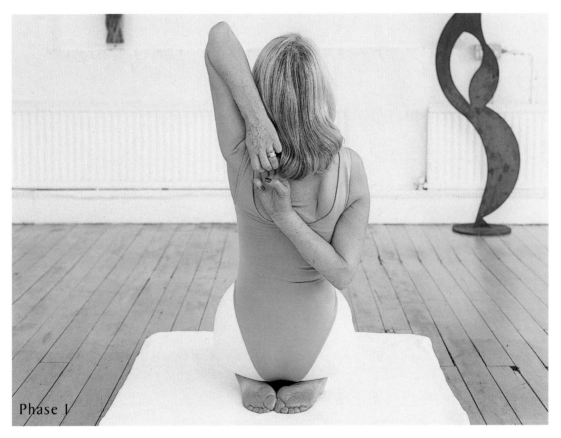

Phase 1

- Sit on your heels (use a cushion as above if this is not yet comfortable for you). Inhale deeply and lift your right arm in the air, then drop it back over your right shoulder.
- Take your left arm up and behind your back and try to join both arms together. Hold your maximum position in this movement for a count of 5. (Don't worry if your hands are still a long way apart; with practice this will improve.)

- Unclasp your hands, relax and repeat on the other side and please notice if you find it easier on one side and difficult on the other. These imbalances can be caused by many things, including heavy shoulder bags that can weigh down one shoulder, or constant use of the right arm as opposed to the left one. The imbalances are important and this movement is invaluable as it will rebalance your shoulders.

  It is also an excellent movement for the lungs, as it helps to open them fully.

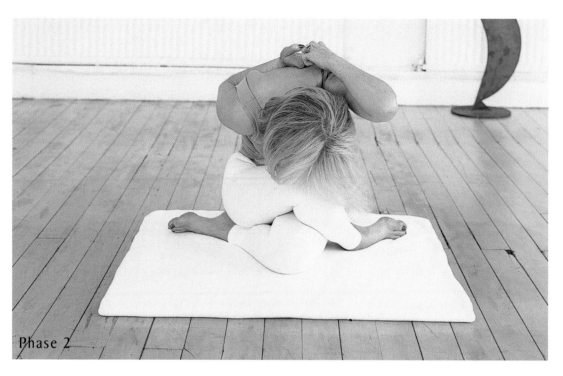

Phase 2

Once you can sit with ease in a kneeling position with your bottom on your heels, then you may try the full posture.

• In a high kneeling position, place your hands on the floor. Cross your right leg over your left and ensure that your heels are hip-width apart.

• Inhale, then, as you exhale and keeping your weight on your hands, carefully lower your bottom between your heels, aiming to sit comfortably in this position. Place your hands on your upper knee and relax. If you can't yet manage this position, don't worry, just repeat Phase 1.

• Sitting in this position, inhale and lift your right arm in the air, take your left one back behind your back and try to clasp them together. Then exhale and bend forwards, aiming your head towards touching your upper knee. Hold this position, breathing normally, for a count of 8. Then inhale and return to an upright position. Exhale, relax and repeat to the other side.

Again, please note that the leg movement may be much easier one side than the other.

'I have been going to Barbara's classes for a few years now and although I'm in my early 50s, I'm more supple and flexible now than in my younger years. I wish I'd started yoga sooner – but I suppose better late than never!'

VERONICA, 51

3   Chest Expansion

This movement relieves tension in the neck and shoulders and can ease the proverbial 'pain in the neck'. It firms and tones the upper arms, corrects posture and firms and tones the muscles that support the bust. As tension in the back of the neck is a frequent cause of headaches, this movement is a boon to headache sufferers.

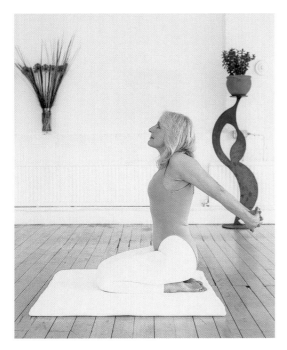

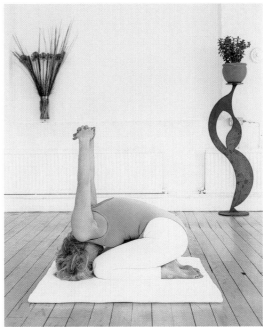

- Sit on your heels with your back straight. Interlock your hands behind your back, ensuring that your elbows are straight. Inhale and lift your arms as high as possible behind your back.

- Exhale and, slowly and carefully, lean forwards, aiming your head to the floor in front of your knees. Hold for a count of 5, breathing normally. Inhale and slowly lift your head and arms. Gradually return to a sitting position, keeping your arms as high as possible. Exhale, slowly lower your arms and relax. Repeat twice.

    On relaxing your arms, you may feel a beautiful warm glow across your shoulders as your muscles relax.

4   Head of a Horse

Many of my desk-bound pupils use this movement to release shoulder tension due to an overload of work at the computer. It is an excellent aid to the prevention of Repetitive Strain Injury (RSI). It also firms the jaw and throat and the muscles that support the bust, and is excellent for retaining the flexibility in the shoulders, elbows, wrists and fingers. Phase 2 increases the flexibility of your hips, knees and ankles and tones your inner thighs.

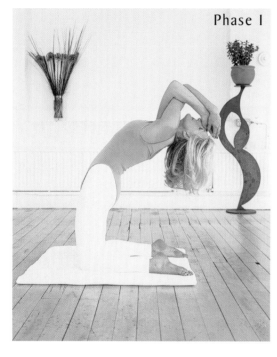

Phase 1

Phase 2

- In a high kneeling position, take your right upper arm over your left, then under the left lower arm and place your palms of your hands together with the thumbs towards your face.
- Now place the first joint of your thumb in the hollow above your nose and between your eyebrows. Inhale deeply and with a full lung, relax backwards, exhaling in your maximum position. Hold your maximum movement for a count of 5, breathing normally.
- Inhale and slowly return to an upright position. Exhale, relax and repeat on the other side. Repeat the entire sequence once.

Only when you can manage Phase 1 with ease, try Phase 2.
- In an all-fours position, place your right foot on your left thigh. Keep your weight on your hands, then place your right knee on the floor. Gently try to come into an upright position, standing on your knees.
- Now entwine your arms together as in Phase 1 and gently bend backwards (please note you will not be able to go as far as in Phase 1). Hold for a count of 5.
- Inhale and return to an upright position, exhale, relax and repeat on the other side. Repeat the entire sequence.

5   Finger Exercises

These movements increase flexibility in the fingers and shoulders, and tone and firm the upper arms. They are excellent and give you super, supple fingers. I really recommend them to people who do a lot of sewing, computer work or who play musical instruments.

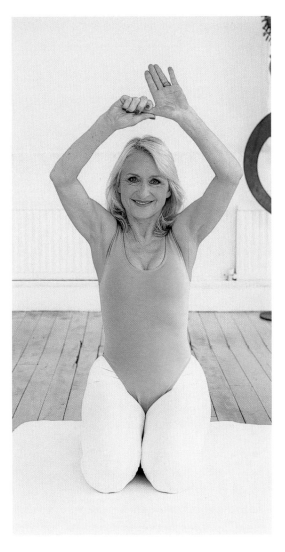

- Sit with your back straight in a kneeling position. Gently massage your hands to warm them. Clasp your left thumb in your right hand and gently pull it slightly.
- Inhale and lift your left thumb in the air, stretching it up as high as possible. Open your elbows as wide as possible, still stretching out your thumb, and lower your hands to your lap.
- Repeat with your first finger and continue until you have exercised all the fingers of this hand, then repeat with the other hand. Massage your hands and then interlock them together, turn them 'inside out', inhale and stretch your arms upwards into the Pose of a Mountain (page 100), hold for a count of 5, then slowly lower your arms and relax.

6 Sideways Body Raise

We first tried this movement in Stage 6. I now repeat it for your convenience.

This is an excellent movement for firming and toning the upper arms, stretching out tension in the wrist and hands and strengthening the arms, helping to prevent osteoporosis. When we fall it is an automatic response to extend a hand or arm to break the fall. If the arms are weak, this can easily lead to a strain or fracture.

Please note: If you have recently had an arm injury, then follow the directions below but *do not lift your body from the floor*. Just put a little weight on your arms and wait until you have regained your strength before moving on to the full movement.

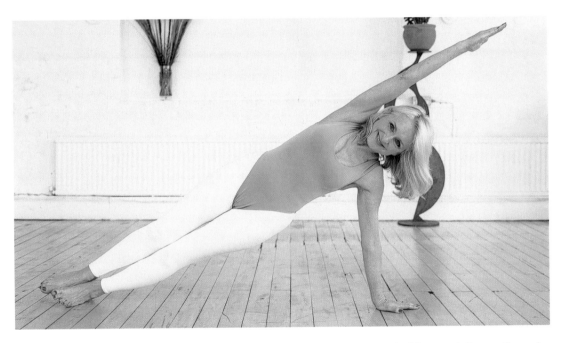

- Sit with both hands to the right side of your body, making sure that both your hands and feet are on a firm, non-slip surface. Bend your knees. Inhale deeply and, as you exhale, lift your body from the floor and support it on both hands and feet.
- Now adjust your body so that your right shoulder is directly above your right wrist and your arm is straight. Lift your bottom and adjust your feet so that the left foot is placed on top of the right one and your body is now in a straight line. When and only when you

feel strong enough, lift your left arm from the floor and stretch it in a straight line, with the inside of your left arm alongside your left ear. Concentrate on a spot on the floor to help your balance, and hold the movement for a count of 5, breathing normally.

- Gently lower your bottom to the floor and relax, then repeat on the other side. Do the movement just once to begin with, but when you feel strong enough then perform the movement twice on each side.

7 Pose of a Plane

We first tried this movement in Stage 5. I am repeating it here for your convenience. A beautiful movement to tone, firm and strengthen the arms, wrists and hands and release lower back tension.

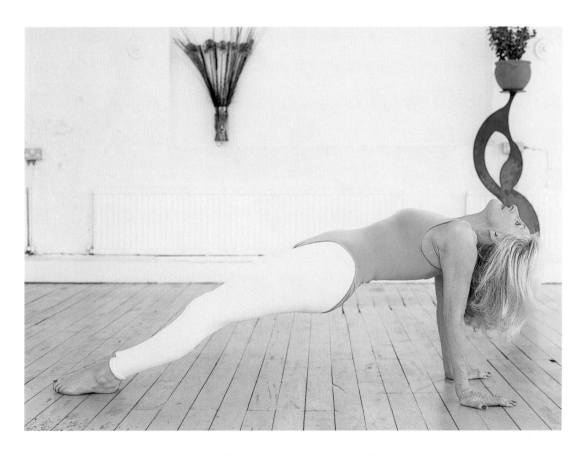

- Sit straight with your hands comfortably on the floor behind you, with your fingertips facing backwards and your legs straight out on the floor in front of you. Ensure that both your hands and feet are on a non-slip surface.
- Inhale deeply and gently lift your body from the floor, supporting your weight on your hands and your feet. Ensure that your body is in a straight line and that your toes are on the floor. Allow your head to drop back and hold your maximum position, breathing normally, for a count of 5, increasing to 10 with practice.
- Slowly lower your body to the floor, relax and repeat once.

8   Pose of a Crow

An excellent arm-strengthener and firmer which also teaches balance and concentration. This movement is quite tricky, so please go carefully, making sure you have a thick blanket in front of you just in case you topple over in your initial attempts.

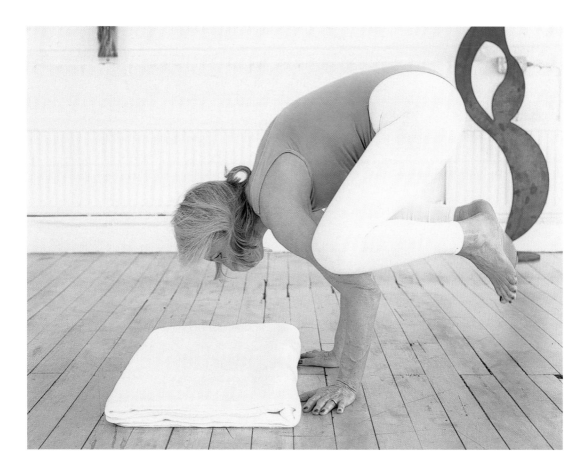

- With your blanket in front of you and on a non-slip surface, spread your hands and fingers out so that your fingers are wide apart (like crow's feet) and position them on the floor in front of you about 1 foot apart.
- Concentrate on a spot in front of you, inhale deeply and, as you exhale, position your knees on the outer portion of your upper arms, keeping your head up. Practise just the above position for a few times and, only when you feel ready, aim to lift your feet from the floor.

- Hold only for a count of 1 to begin with, then gradually and carefully build it up until you are holding for a count of 10. Then lower your feet to the floor and relax and repeat once. (Please don't feel a failure if this feels almost impossible at first – it is difficult for all of us, but fantastic when you finally manage it – and with practice you will. I promise!)

9   Pose of Eight Curves

This is another hand-balance and yes, it is difficult at first, but you do want to look and feel younger, and arms are a huge give-away. Don't give up, just keep practising and I guarantee that you will be delighted with your firm, toned and beautiful arms and you will find your concentration and balance improving tremendously as well!

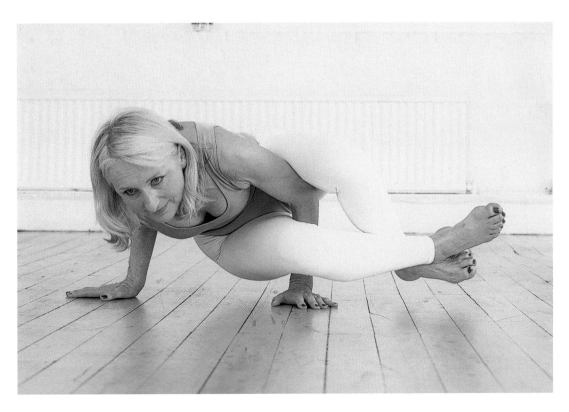

- Sit on the floor with your legs in front of you. Bend your knees and cross your right leg over your left.
- Now take your left hand under your right knee and place it on the floor. Place your right hand on the floor about 1 foot from the left. Bend your elbows and lower your body near to the floor, with your chin just 3 inches from the floor. Inhale deeply and, as you exhale, try to lift your body off the floor, balancing on just your hands.

- Hold for a count of 1 to begin with, increasing to 10 with practice. To come out of the position, gently lower your body to the floor, relax and repeat on the other side.

   Please note that in this movement, it is normal to find one side much easier than the other. It is just another case of yoga rebalancing the body.

Please do not
attempt if you
are pregnant

10 Pose of an Elephant

This is quite difficult to begin with, but tones and strengthens your arms and is a great toner for your thighs.

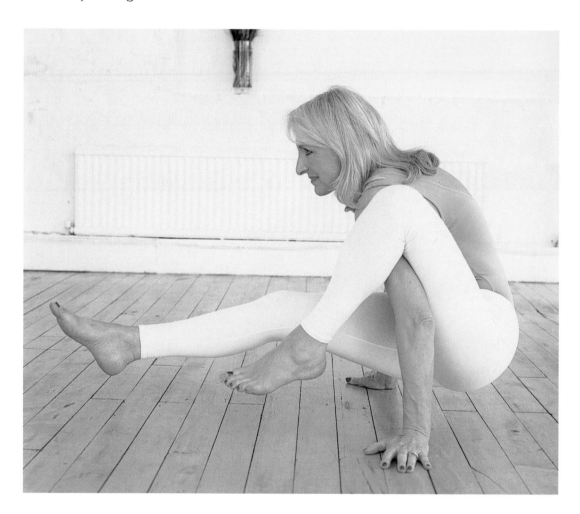

- Sit straight with both legs straight out in front of you. Carefully lift your right leg as high as possible over your right upper arm. Keep your left leg straight and place your hands by your hips with your fingers pointing forwards.
- Inhale deeply and, as you exhale, leaning forwards, balancing on your hands and keeping your left leg straight, aim to lift your

bottom and left leg from the floor. Hold for a count of 3 to start with, increasing to 5 with practice. Gently lower your bottom and leg to the floor and then repeat on the other side.
- Do not repeat as this movement is very strong and it is better to rebuild your strength carefully and gradually.

11 Pose of a Firefly

This is such a lovely balance, however it helps tremendously to be able to do the Pose of a Tortoise (Stage 6, page 78) prior to trying this movement, as it needs flexibility in both the hips and lower back.

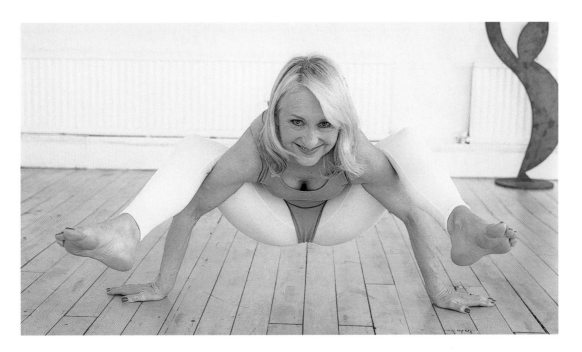

- Sit straight with your legs straight out in front of you. Bend your legs so that your feet and knees are about 1 foot apart.
- Inhale and place your hands in prayer, then lower your elbows towards the floor between your knees. Now take your hands under your legs so that your elbows are on *the outer side of your knees*. (If you can't manage to have your elbows on the outer side of your knees at

this stage, then keep practising, but do not attempt the rest of this movement until this is possible.)

- Lean forwards and stretch your arms back a little, then gently lift your bottom and legs from the floor and balance on your hands, breathing normally. Hold for a count of 5, then gently lower your bottom to the floor and relax. Repeat once.

'After a severe head injury I was left paralysed on the right-hand side of my body. My balance and co-ordination were very poor. Having taken up yoga three years ago, my mobility and flexibility have improved far more than I thought possible. Not only am I fitter and healthier now, I am more focused on things that matter and with Barbara's encouragement, I'm sure that I will achieve even more.'

SUSAN, 55

12 Relaxation

Following the above movement, lie flat on your back and relax each muscle in turn. Slow your breathing down and concentrate on your slow, calm exhalations. Relax your body totally.

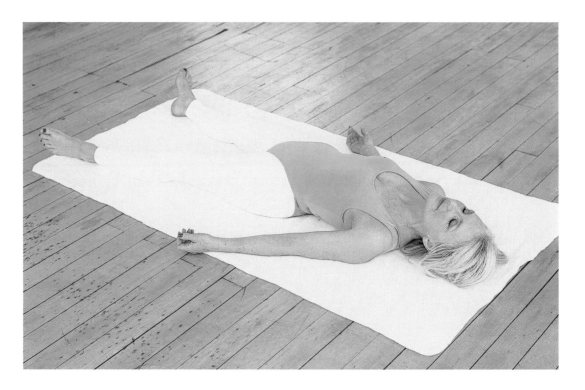

Flat Stomach Plan

These movements do wonders for your midriff, waistline and abdominals. Every single one of them has been fully explained earlier, so you have already practised these movements and become familiar with them. I am therefore giving you this chapter in a chart form, so that if this area of your body is a particular challenge (and it normally is), you can practise these movements as well as, or instead of, your 15-minute plans.

Caution: **Remember to go carefully and without any strain at all. Please do not attempt any of these movements if you are pregnant.**

❛ To love oneself is the beginning of a lifelong romance. ❜
OSCAR WILDE

Flat Stomach Plan

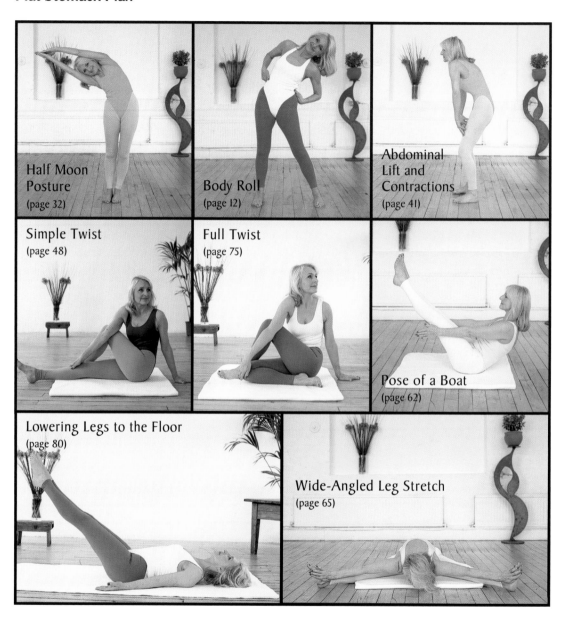

Half Moon Posture (page 32)

Body Roll (page 12)

Abdominal Lift and Contractions (page 41)

Simple Twist (page 48)

Full Twist (page 75)

Pose of a Boat (page 62)

Lowering Legs to the Floor (page 80)

Wide-Angled Leg Stretch (page 65)

At the end of your flat stomach plan, draw your knees to your chest and rock your back gently from side to side then lie down, slow down your breathing and relax your entire body, focusing on a lovely feeling of peace and calm. Relaxation is described fully on page 57.

Bottom, Hips and Thighs

My personal belief is that yoga is the best exercise system ever for streamlining these areas. I have witnessed so many pupils start in class with sagging bottoms, jodhpur thighs and a massive amount of cellulite that no miracle lotion or potion had been able to dissolve, but after doing their yoga these problem areas just gradually disappeared, giving them slim, sleek, perfectly toned hips and thighs.

These movements will be familiar to you, as all of them have been described earlier in this book. I have made two charts for you – one a.m. chart and one p.m. chart – which again may be done as well as or instead of your 15-Minute Miracles stretches. The results will be fantastic.

❛No woman should ever be quite accurate about her age.
It looks so calculating.❜

OSCAR WILDE

Bottom, Hips and Thigh Plan (a.m.)

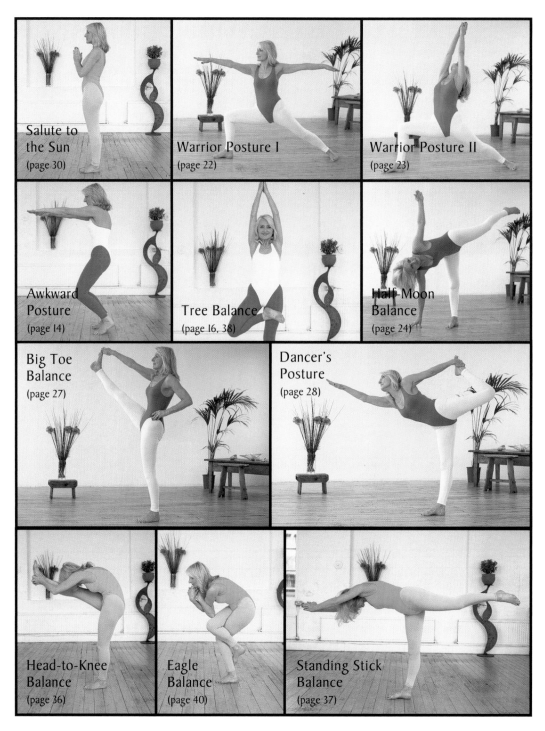

Salute to the Sun (page 30)

Warrior Posture I (page 22)

Warrior Posture II (page 23)

Awkward Posture (page 14)

Tree Balance (page 16, 38)

Half-Moon Balance (page 24)

Big Toe Balance (page 27)

Dancer's Posture (page 28)

Head-to-Knee Balance (page 36)

Eagle Balance (page 40)

Standing Stick Balance (page 37)

At the end of these movements, draw your knees to your chest, interlock your hands around them and rock your lower back from side to side. Then lie flat, slow down your breathing and gently relax your body (see page 57).

Bottom, Hips and Thigh Plan (p.m.)

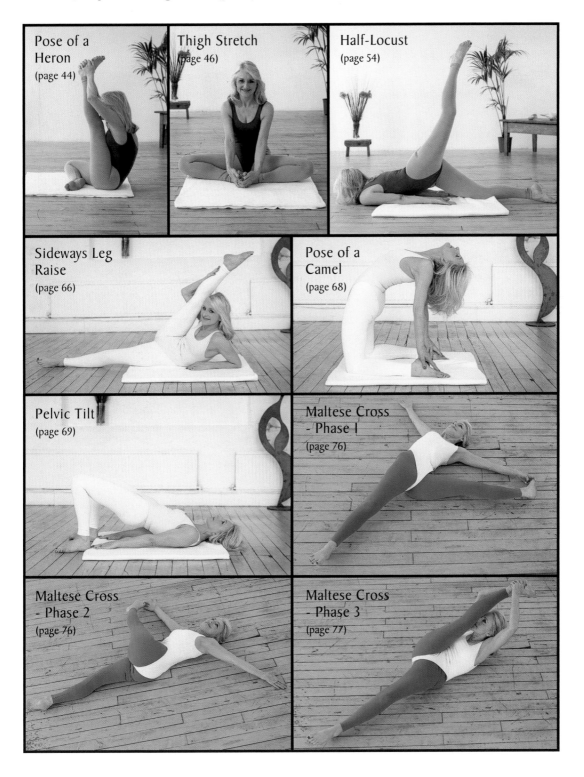

Pose of a Heron (page 44)

Thigh Stretch (page 46)

Half-Locust (page 54)

Sideways Leg Raise (page 66)

Pose of a Camel (page 68)

Pelvic Tilt (page 69)

Maltese Cross - Phase 1 (page 76)

Maltese Cross - Phase 2 (page 76)

Maltese Cross - Phase 3 (page 77)

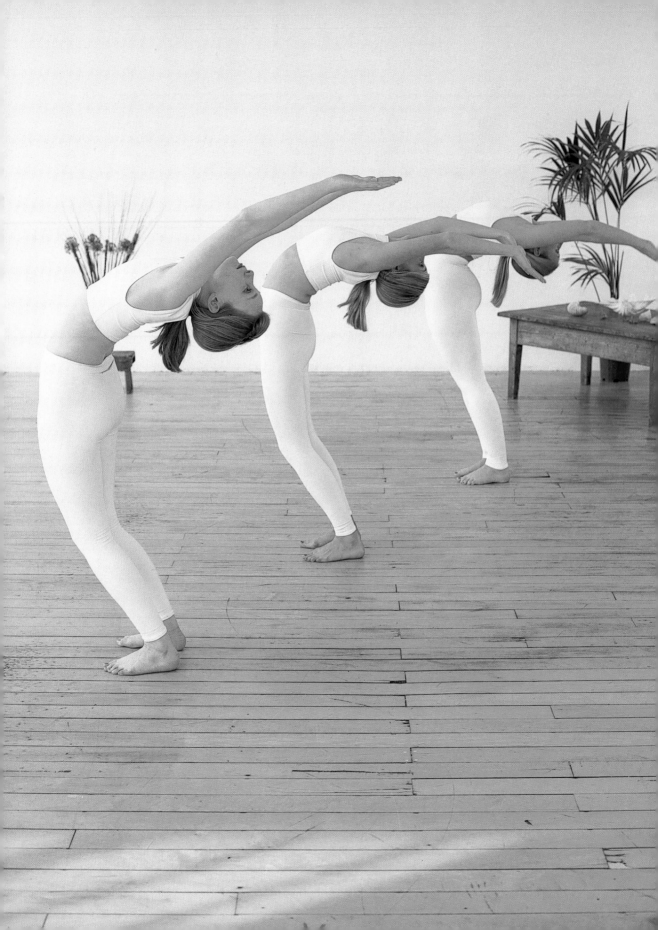

Your Ageless Body

I hope that by now you have kept to your 15-minutes-per-day commitment and are reaping yoga's incredible benefits. So if you are ready, let's move on from 15 years younger to ageless agility.

- Salute to the Sun
- Intense Sideways Stretch
- The Wheel
- Pose of a Monkey
- The Advanced Twist
- Alternate Leg Pull with Foot Clasp
- The Lotus Position
- Pose of the Scales
- Pose of a Cowherd
- Slow-Motion Firming
- Relaxation and Relaxing Breath

The most beautiful makeup of a woman is passion, but cosmetics are easier to buy.

YVES SAINT LAURENT

1 Salute to the Sun

When you first started this I bet you found both the synchronization and the movements in this sequence very difficult to do. By now, however, your body should be much more agile, and eventually it will be second nature for you to get up in the morning and perform this brilliant energizing sequence with effortless ease. When you feel able, do it as shown, with your feet together.

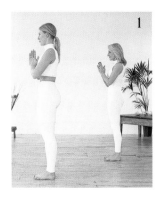

- Stand straight with your feet together, perfect posture and hands in prayer. Inhale slowly and deeply, then calmly exhale.

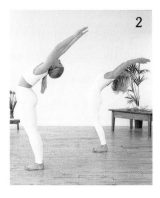

- Inhale and lift your arms up above your head. Gently bend backwards, exhaling in your maximum position.

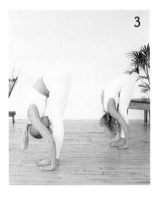

- Inhale and slowly return to an upright position, exhale and, with your head up, back flat and legs straight, gently bend forwards and place your hands on the floor by your feet.

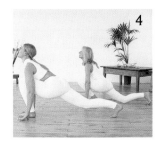

- Inhale and stretch your right leg backwards. Look upwards.

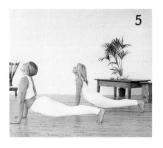

- Exhale and take your left leg backwards.

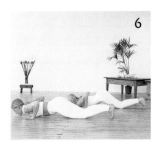

- Place your knees on the floor first, then your chest and then your chin.

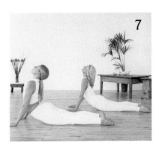

- Inhale and slowly lift your upper body into Cobra position.

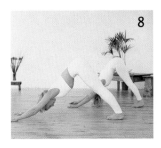

- Exhale as you lift your bottom in the air and stretch your heels and head towards the floor, moving your body into an inverted 'V' position.

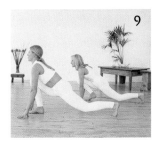

- Inhale as you place your right foot between your hands and look upwards.

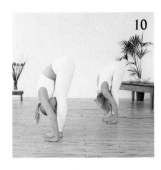

- Exhale as you bring your left leg between your hands. Now lift your bottom in the air and aim to straighten your legs.

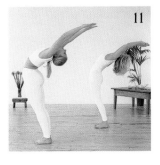

- Inhale deeply, lift both your head and your arms and gently come up into an upright position. Gently bend backwards in your maximum backwards bend.

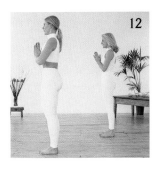

- Inhale as you return to an upright position, place your hands together in prayer and relax. Repeat the entire sequence, this time taking the left leg back first in positions 4 and 9.

2   Intense Sideways Stretch

This movement corrects poor posture and stiffness in the shoulders and wrists. It releases tightness in the chest and increases the elasticity of the hip joints and spine.

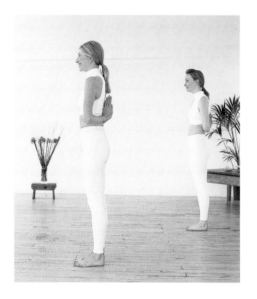

• Stand straight with your feet together and place your hands in prayer behind your back. Carefully turn your hands upwards so that they are in prayer behind your back with your fingers pointing to your head.

   Please note: I have noticed that some pupils find the above movement incredibly easy, whilst others find this wrist and hand movement almost impossible. If you are one of the latter, try this movement gently and carefully without strain. If it is too difficult for you, then just fold your arms behind your back until your wrists are sufficiently flexible to place them in prayer.

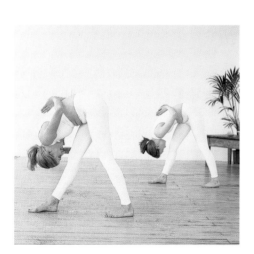

• Place your legs 3½–4 feet apart, and inhale deeply. As you exhale, turn your right foot 90 degrees to the right, keeping your left foot facing forwards. Turn to face over your right foot, inhale deeply and, as you exhale, gently and slowly bend forwards, aiming your chin towards your shin. Relax in your maximum position without strain and hold for a count of 5, increasing to 10 as you progress in the position. Inhale and slowly return to an upright position, exhale, relax and repeat to the left-hand side. Once you have performed the movement on both sides, stand straight, correct your posture and, still keeping your hands together in prayer behind your back, aim to press your hands hard together. Hold for a count of 5, then slowly and carefully undo your hands. Massage your wrists and relax, then repeat the entire sequence once.

3 The Wheel

This really does give you that energized, ageless body! It gives the spine tremendous flexibility and agility. As most of us did it in childhood, it literally brings back our youth! It strengthens the arms, wrists and fingers and relieves tension in the shoulders and lower back, and is a most wonderful energizing stretch. It stimulates blood flow to the spinal nerves and helps to prevent degeneration of the spine.

Because some people never managed the movement in childhood and others have had a long gap since they last practised it, please take care.

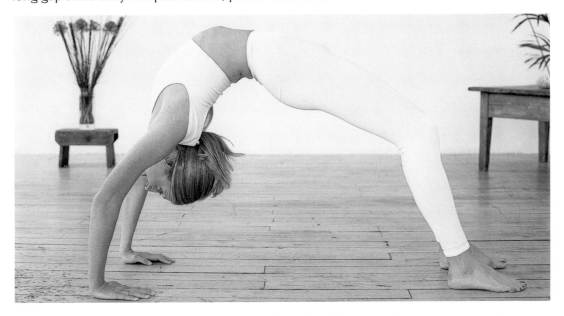

- Lie flat on your back, bend your knees and draw your feet towards your body so that your heels are flat on the floor, hip-distance apart and your fingertips can just touch them when your arms are by your sides.
- Now take your hands back and place them at shoulder level with your fingertips pointing towards your feet and the heels of your hands flat on the floor. (Note: this can be very difficult at first due to stiffness in the shoulders, don't give up but don't continue with the movement until you can place your hands in this position with ease.)
- Now, with your feet and hands in the correct position, inhale deeply and push down on your hands, aiming to lift your entire body from the

floor. This may take many attempts, but eventually with practice it will happen. Once you are in your maximum stretch, exhale and hold just for a count of 1 to begin with, building up to a count of 10 as you progress in the movement. Breathe normally in your maximum position, eventually aiming to straighten both your arms and your legs.
- Gently lower your whole body to the floor and relax. Do not repeat until the movement becomes easy for you, and then do it twice. Well done – now, doesn't this make you feel years younger?! Draw your knees to your chest and rock from side to side. Lie flat on the floor, relax and take 10 slow, calm, deep breaths.

4   Pose of a Monkey

You may think that you will never manage this movement, but with daily practice you will – and when you do you will feel fantastic. Mentally it opens new horizons as you think that, having mastered this seemingly difficult movement, then what else is possible? Physically it relieves lower back tension and can help sciatica sufferers. It is great for toning and firming your thighs and increasing the flexibility of your hamstrings. With your new flexibility in your lower back, your walk will look 15 years younger.

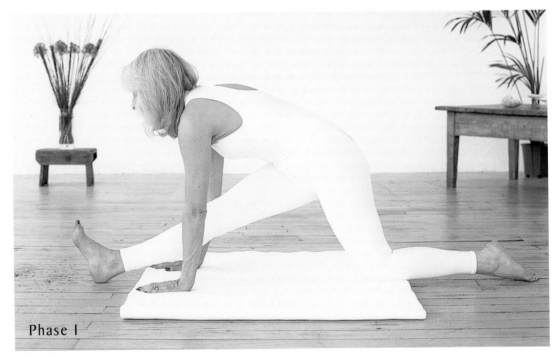

Phase 1

- Kneel on your mat with your knees about 1 foot apart. Place your hands on the floor in front of you, directly under your shoulders and about 1 foot apart. Stretch your right leg out in front of you and ensure that your hands are either side of your right leg and are supporting your weight. Hold your maximum stretch for a count of 5 without straining, then gently draw your leg back again and relax.

'I started going to yoga classes seven years ago with my mum, who'd been referred by her doctor because of back problems. I used to go to the gym five times a week, but as I get the most benefit out of yoga I decided to stop going to the gym. For me, the main benefits are stress relief and relaxation, but the thing I love about yoga is that it's a total body workout, both inside and out. I've been doing it for so long now that I can't imagine giving it up!'

JULIE, 26

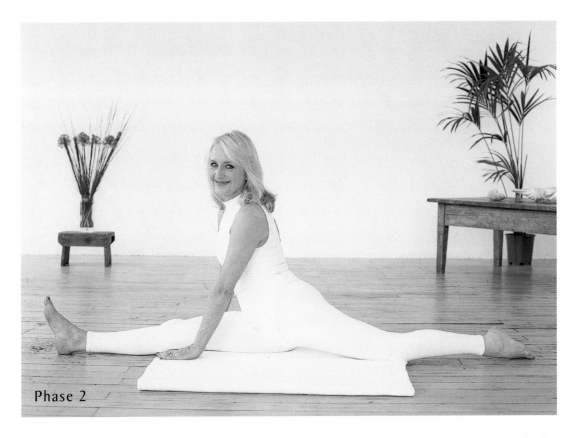

Phase 2

- Now, keeping your weight on your hands, inhale deeply. As you exhale, stretch your right foot forwards as far as possible without strain. Hold your maximum position for a count of 5, then slowly draw your right leg back to a kneeling position, relax and repeat to the other side. Repeat the entire sequence once.

Help and Advice
It takes quite a while to master the full movement. Please don't be put off if your early attempts seem very feeble. You really will master this stretch with gentle daily practice without strain.

5   The Advanced Twist

This movement creates amazing flexibility in the spine and can help relieve lower back ache, lumbago and hip pains. It is excellent for increasing the flexibility of the neck and shoulders, and tones and firms the midriff, waistline, hips and throat. It helps to prevent sluggishness in both the spleen and liver.

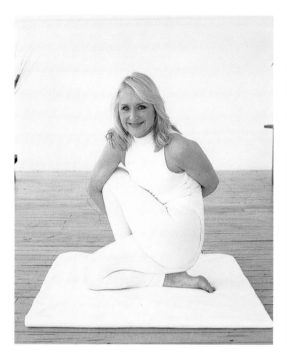

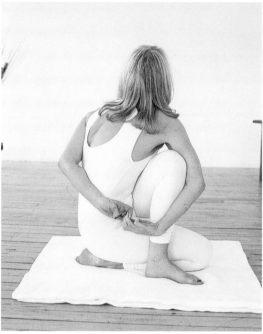

- Sit straight with both legs straight out in front of you. Bring your right foot into the space between your thighs and carefully sit on it so your right heel is under your right buttock.
- Place your left hand on the floor behind your back. Place your left foot on the floor on the outer side of your right thigh. Take your right arm around your left knee and take your left arm behind your back and try to join them,

eventually clasping them together. Correct your posture and turn your head over your left shoulder.
- Hold for a count of 5 to begin with, increasing to 10 as you progress in the movement. To come out of the position, slowly bring your head forwards, unclasp your hands and return to a sitting position. Repeat to the other side. Repeat the entire sequence once.

'Although I have always exercised and tried to keep healthy and fit, it wasn't until I discovered yoga that everything fell into place. Barbara is a complete inspiration to me. Although I still have a very long way to go, it really is worth the effort, for every day I feel more supple, more balanced, relaxed and healthy. What more could one hope for?'

MONIQUE, 60

6 Alternate Leg Pull with Foot Clasp

We practised the beginner stage of this movement in Stage 4. Now, if you are ready, let's try to move on a little.

This movement will stretch your hamstrings and spine and keep your knees, ankles and hips flexible, and tone your abdominal organs. The extra arm clasp is excellent for toning the arms, removing tension in the shoulders and correcting drooping shoulders.

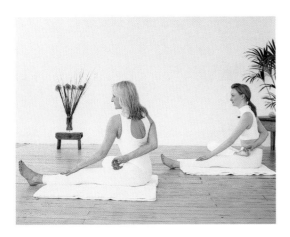

- Sit straight with both legs straight out in front of you. Inhale and lift your right foot onto your left thigh. Exhale and gently take your right hand behind your back and aim to grab your right foot. (If this is not yet possible, keep your foot on your upper thigh if it feels comfortable – if not, place it in the space between your legs and place both arms parallel to your left leg.)

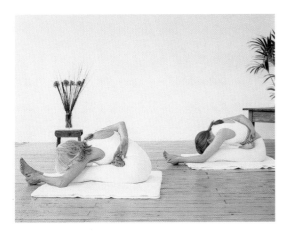

- Inhale and, as you exhale, gently stretch forwards to grab your left foot and gently draw your chin towards your shin. Hold your maximum position for a count of 10, breathing normally, then inhale and return to an upright position. Exhale, relax and repeat on the other side. If you can clasp your right foot in your right hand, inhale deeply and, as you exhale, gently stretch forwards clasping your left foot in your left hand and aiming your chin towards your shin, still keeping your right foot clasped behind your back. Hold your maximum position for a count of 10, breathing normally. Inhale and return to an upright position, exhale, unclasp your foot, relax and repeat on the other side. Repeat the entire sequence once.

Help and Advice
You may find it much easier to clasp your foot on one side than the other. This is quite normal, and just another movement that yoga uses to realign and balance our bodies. With practice you will be able to do it on both sides.

7   The Lotus Position

This movement is one of yoga's most famous sitting positions. The back is straight in this position, so keeping the mind alert, and it restores the flexibility of the knees, hips and ankles. Because the legs are locked in this position it is impossible to fidget. It is used for many breathing exercises and for meditation.

Regaining the necessary flexibility can take a while, but once you can do it, it honestly is both comfortable and relaxing. Even when you can do this movement with ease, I always advise pupils to loosen up their legs prior to starting the position.

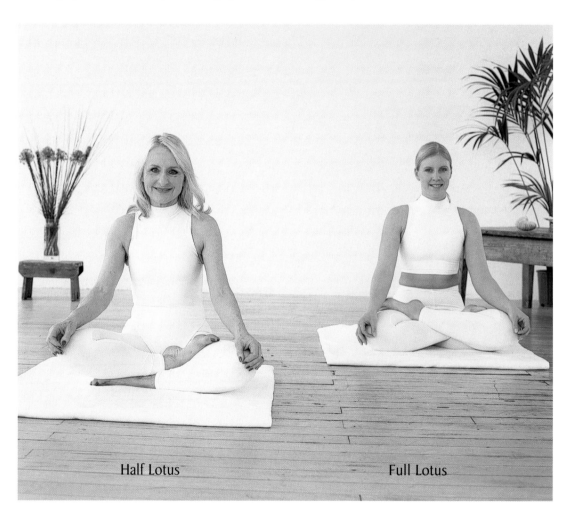

Half Lotus   Full Lotus

- Sit straight with both legs straight out in front of you.
- Inhale and lift your right foot onto your left thigh, and gently place your hand on your right knee. Exhale and gently bounce your right knee towards the floor 5 times, then relax and repeat this loosening and warming-up movement with your left foot.
- Once you feel that your legs are sufficiently loosened up, then try the lotus positions.

Half Lotus

- In a sitting position with your legs straight out in front of you, gently place your right foot in the space between your legs with your heel towards your groin.
- Carefully lift your left foot onto your right thigh. Sit comfortably in this position with your back straight, breathing slowly and deeply and holding the movement for 5 slow, deep breaths. Gently remove your left foot from your right thigh and perform the movement the other way round.

Full Lotus

Only attempt this when the Half-Lotus is really comfortable.

- Sit straight with both legs stretched out in front of you.
- Breathe in deeply, and gently place your right foot on your left thigh. Now, very carefully, try to place your left foot on your right thigh. This could take very many attempts – don't worry and don't strain. Hold this position for 5 very slow, deep breaths, and then carefully take your feet out of this position, relax and massage them and then repeat the movement, this time placing your left foot on your right thigh first. It is really important to alternate your legs in this posture, to ensure correct balance of the flexibility in your ankles, hips and knees (most people start with one side much more flexible than the other).

Movements in the Lotus Position

Once you can do the Lotus Position with ease, it is great to move on and do some of the many postures in the Lotus Position.

Help and Advice

Please note that when you do manage this movement for the first time it is nearly always most uncomfortable. However, with practice it does become both very comfortable and very relaxing.

8 Pose of the Scales

This is extremely beneficial for stretching out the wrists and strengthening the arms and hands.

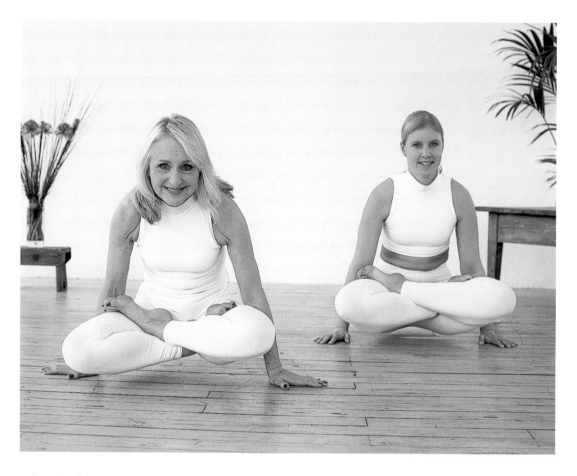

- Sit in Full Lotus position and place your hands by your hips.
- Take a deep breath in and, as you exhale, transfer your weight to your hands and aim to lift your body from the floor, balancing on just your hands.

- Hold for a count of 5 at first, increasing to 10 as your strength improves. Slowly lower your bottom to the floor, undo your legs and relax.

'I joined Barbara's classes one year after a major spine operation. I couldn't walk properly or drive. Within a few months I was mobile again. I went on to do a trek in the Amazon forest.'

IRENE, 70

9   Pose of a Cowherd

This gives you all the benefits of the Lotus position and greatly improves your sense of balance. It is not easy, but you feel so good when you have achieved it.

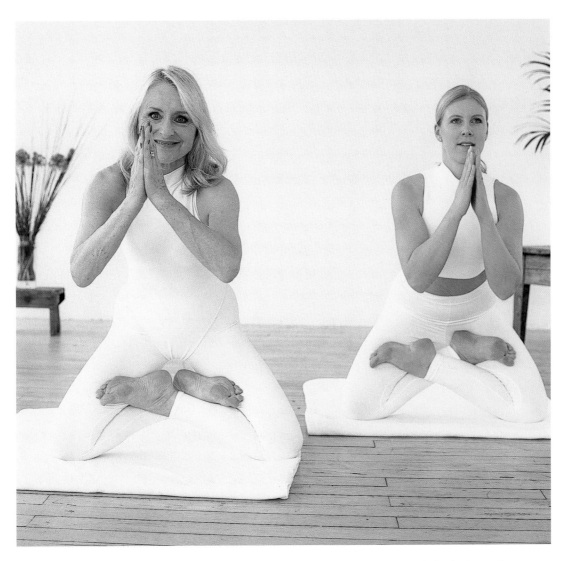

- Sit in the Full Lotus position on a very thick mat.
- Take a deep breath in and place your hands on the floor in front of you.
- Concentrate on a spot to help you balance and gradually lift your upper body into a vertical position so that you are balancing on your knees. Now, when fully balanced, aim to remain upright and place your hands together in prayer. Try to hold for a count of 5 and then relax, lower your bottom to the floor, undo your legs and massage your knees, feet and ankles, then repeat with your legs the other way round. Well done!

10 Slow-Motion Firming

This is a lovely, relaxing sequence to remove all tension from your spine and give you a fantastic, firm, flat, strong, beautifully toned tummy. It can be done at any time, but is especially good to do before you go to sleep at night.

There are no holds, just do it in a slow continuous motion.

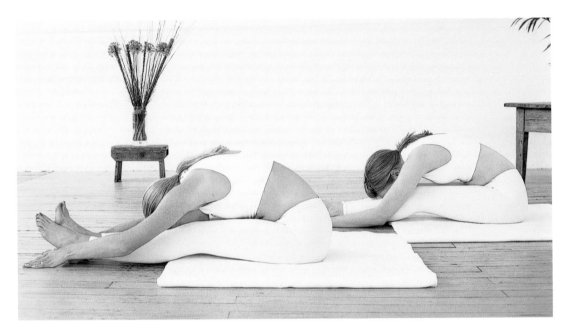

• Sit up with your back straight and both legs stretched out in front of you. Inhale slowly and deeply. Exhale as you slowly move forwards into Backstretch, keeping your head up and your back straight. Aim eventually to clasp your feet and draw your head to your knees.

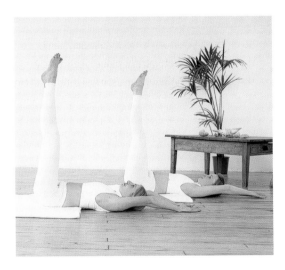

• Inhale as you slowly return to an upright position. Exhale as you slowly and gently lie flat on your back and take your arms straight back behind your head. Bend your knees, inhale and lift your legs so they are at right angles to the floor.

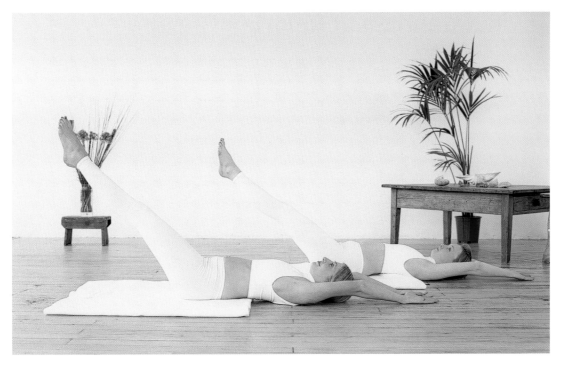

- Exhale as you slowly lower your legs to the floor, keeping them straight. To begin with, make this part of the movement a little faster than normal, to make it easy for you – you can slow it down when both your back and abdomen become stronger. (Please note: for people with weak backs and stomach muscles it is not unusual to experience a small pull in the lower back as you lower your legs to the floor. If this is the case, then bend your knees as soon as this happens and continue to lower your legs to the floor with them bent. Each time you practise the movement, aim to get a little further before you have to bend your knees. Eventually, when you are stronger, you will be able to lower them to the floor keeping them straight the whole time.)

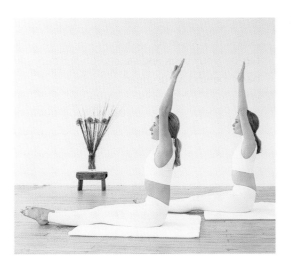

- Inhale as you come into a sitting position, stretching your arms up in the air. (If you find this difficult, then gently place your elbows on the floor to help you push up into a sitting position.) Exhale as you once more relax forward into a Backstretch. You have now performed one whole cycle. Repeat 4 times. You will feel very relaxed and your results – a firm, flat, beautifully toned tummy – will be visible very soon. Congratulations.

11 Relaxation and Relaxing Breath

Following this sequence, it is now lovely to lie flat and relax.

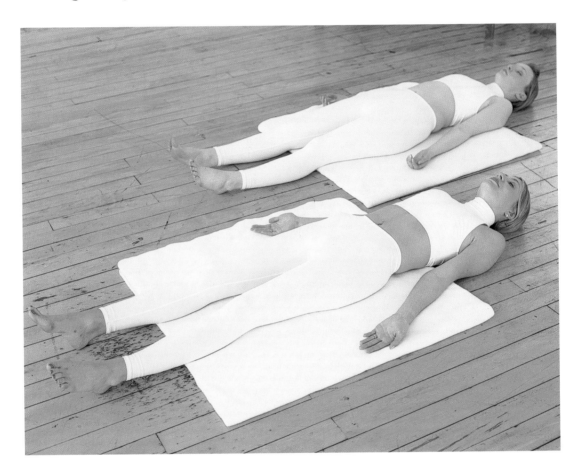

- Slowly relax all your muscles in turn and close your eyes and now relax body and mind with the relaxing breath.
- Gently push your abdominals out and inhale for a slow count of 4, hold your breath for a count of 4, and then slowly exhale through your nose for a count of 6.
- Repeat 10 times and relax, relax, relax.

Come away from the din, come away to the quiet fields over which the great sky stretches, and where, between us and the stars, there lies but silence; and there in the stillness let us listen to the voice that is speaking within us.

JEROME K JEROME

Amazing Age-defying Anti-gravity Movements

Caution: **Please do not attempt any of the movements in this chapter if you have high blood pressure or any problems whatsoever with your head or neck area or are pregnant.**

Having got this far in your yoga practice, you should now be feeling very much better. Your body should be feeling great – much stronger and more flexible – so now I have saved the best until last. It is your turn to try yoga's inverted positions. These are incredible: they give you energy and do wonders for your skin, hair, eyesight, hearing and feeling of well-being.

Please note these movements are not arranged in a 15-minute sequence for you to try, and I do not want you to try more than one movement at a time.

Start when you feel ready, the ideal time being when you have just finished one of your 15-minute sequences, and remember these movements are strong so please don't strain.

- Pose of a Peacock

- Peacock in the Lotus Position

- Handstand

- Pose of a Scorpion

- Shoulderstand and Bridge Position

- Pose of Tranquillity in the Lotus Position

- Pose of a Fish in the Lotus Position

- The Wide-Angled Plough

- The Noose

- The Yoga Sleeping Pose

- The Classic Headstand

- Half-Split and Eagle in Headstand

One doesn't discover new lands without consenting to lose sight of the shore for a very long time.
ANDRE GIDE

1   Pose of a Peacock

Please do not attempt if you have high blood pressure

Please do not attempt if you have head or neck problems

Please do not attempt if you are pregnant

This is wonderful, it is very energizing and a great strengthener and toner for your arms and wrists. It gives your arms amazing shape and, as you have to concentrate hard, it is great for clearing the mind. The movement has traditionally been recommended as helpful for diabetes sufferers, as it massages the digestive organs and pancreas.

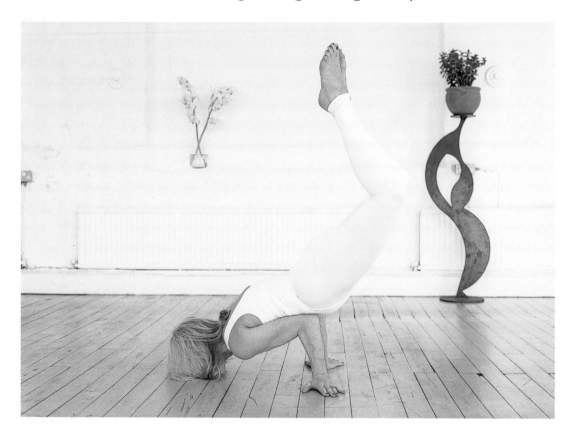

- Kneel on the floor and place your hands on the floor in front of you, as near together as possible, with the fingers pointing either outwards or backwards (I find some pupils have a preference for one way and some for the other).
- Now lunge forwards over your hands so that your elbows are on the inside of your hip-bones, and your chin is just above the floor.

Inhale and, as you exhale, gently lift both your legs in the air and hold your maximum position for a count of 5, then gently lower your legs to the floor and relax.

- For a stronger stretch, place your chin on the floor in your maximum position and lift your legs higher.

Help and Advice
Very few pupils manage this on their first attempt, and most find it extremely difficult. There is very little advice I can give you, except to tell you that with practice you will do it – and once you do manage it you will be so thrilled, it will have been worth the struggle.

LOOK 15 YEARS YOUNGER

2 Peacock in the Lotus Position

This incredible movement has all the benefits of both the Peacock position and the Lotus position (page 128). Please don't attempt it until you can do both these movements with ease.

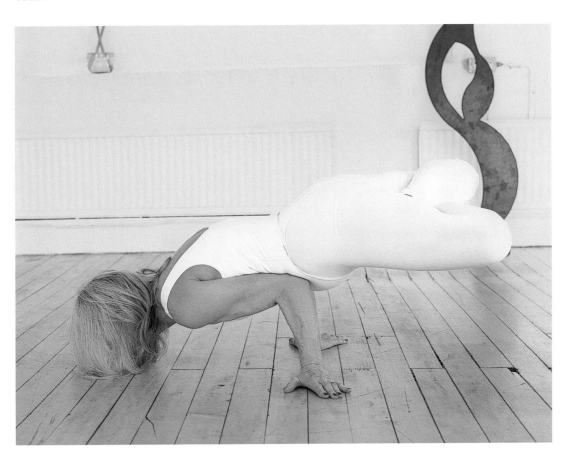

- In a Full Lotus position, come into an 'all fours' position with your weight on your hands and knees.
- Now adjust your hands so that your fingers point either backwards or outwards and your elbows are on the inside of your hipbones. Inhale and, as you exhale, lift your body from the floor.
- Hold for a count of 5, then exhale and relax.

Help and Advice
No, it is not easy, but again it is such a wonderful sense of achievement when you do make it. Isn't it great to be getting younger and more flexible as you get older?

3 Handstand

This literally brings back your youth – most adults haven't done a handstand since childhood, and some not even then, so when I introduce them to it they are a little nervous. On mastering it, however, the effect is amazing, they feel like teenagers again and can't believe the energy it gives them and the amazing shape of their arms. It strengthens the wrists, shoulders and arms, expands the chest and is excellent for the skin, hair and brain cells, due to the increased blood flow in that area.

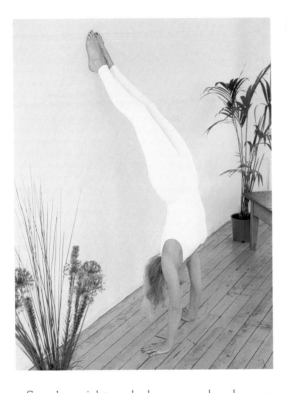
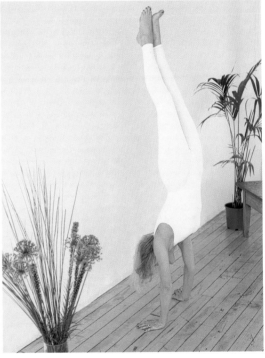

- Stand straight and place your hands on a non-slip surface shoulder-width apart and about 1 foot from a wall. Make sure your arms are straight. Inhale deeply and, as you exhale, aim to lift your legs and swing them up to the wall. When you first start this may resemble a tiny jump, but keep on practising and eventually your feet will reach the wall. As soon as this happens, stay there for a count of 5, then gently lower your legs to the floor, take your bottom to your heels and stay in the Pose of a Swan for a count of 10, to allow your circulation to return to normal.

- When you have gained confidence in the position, when in Full Handstand concentrate on a spot on the floor to assist your balance, take your feet from the wall and try to balance with your toes pointed and your head raised. Please note that once you have gained confidence in the movement it is possible to do the Handstand without the aid of a wall. I do recommend, however, that if you try this movement you have a couple of friends ready to catch you in case of a fall!

4 Pose of a Scorpion

This movement is great for boosting energy and concentration, and fantastic for relieving shoulder tension. It is excellent for strengthening your arms, hands and elbows. This is so rejuvenating you will feel just great after it.

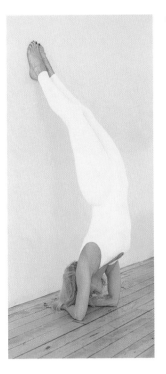

- Kneel on the floor by a wall and place your elbows shoulder-width apart on a non-slip mat. Your thumbs should point towards each other. Keep your head up and, keeping your elbows on the floor, lift your bottom in the air, then inhale and, still keeping your head and arms in this position, kick your legs upwards and aim your feet to touch the wall. This can take quite a few attempts, but just keep persevering. You will feel fantastic when you master it. Hold your maximum position for a count of 5, then gently come out of the position, lower your bottom to your heels, then relax in Pose of a Swan for a count of 5, breathing normally.

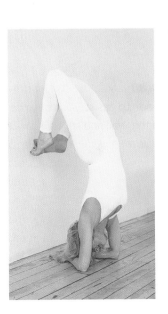

- Once your balance has been secured in full Scorpion position, try to walk your feet down the wall in the direction of your head, and hold this position for a count of 5. These two movements give you an amazing feeling of agility and YOUTH.

  Please note: It is possible to do the Scorpion position from the classical Headstand. I, however, prefer to teach it in the first instance as above, by a wall, with me by my pupil's side so there is no chance of a fall.

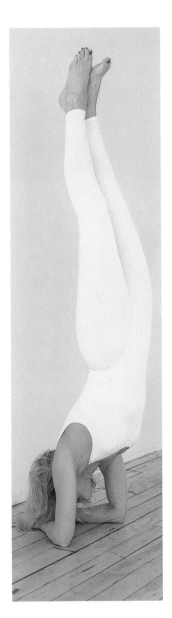

- Once you have mastered the Scorpion, then try to take your feet off the wall and balance.

5 Shoulderstand and Bridge Position

Please do not attempt if you have high blood pressure

Please do not attempt if you have head or neck problems

Please do not attempt if you are pregnant

We first practised the Shoulderstand in Stage 6 (page 83). I do hope that you have been enjoying this magical posture and are now ready to move on to some exciting new movements.

The Shoulderstand and Bridge Position, as well as affording all the benefits of the Shoulderstand, greatly increases the strength and flexibility of the lower back, hands and wrists.

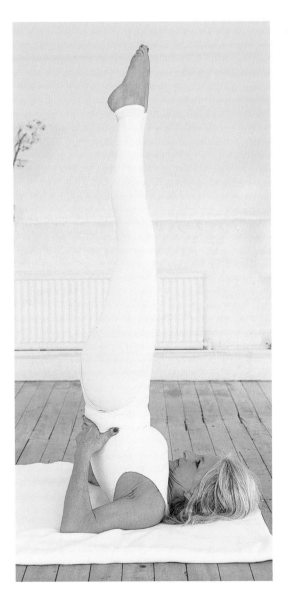

- In a perfect straight Shoulderstand, support your back with your hands at your waistline, your thumbs in front and your fingers behind, pointing towards your feet. Ensure that your fingers are near together and your elbows as near your body as possible.

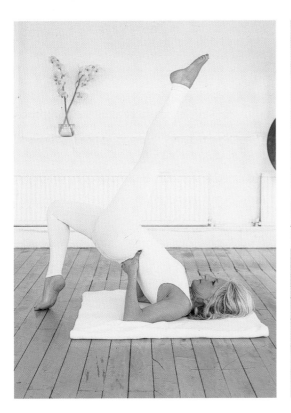

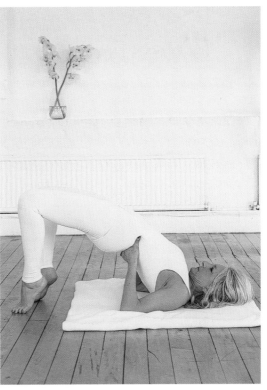

- Gently lower your right leg towards the floor (this looks easy but in fact may take several attempts).

- If your foot touches the floor, then try to drop your left foot down as well. Hold this position for a count of 10, breathing normally, then inhale and lift your legs back up into a Shoulderstand – do this one leg at a time. (This again looks easy but does require a flexible spine, flexible wrists and a very strong lower back. If you find it too difficult in your first attempts, then gently lower your body to the floor and relax.) Come out of this position in exactly the same way as you would for the Shoulderstand. Lie flat on the floor and arch your body into the Pose of a Fish (Stage 6, page 84).

'In the last four years yoga has brought me, mentally, a more controlled outlook on life and, physically, increased flexibility and stamina. I wish I had discovered yoga sooner.'

SARAH, 39

6 Pose of Tranquillity in the Lotus Position

Please do not attempt if you have high blood pressure

Please do not attempt if you have head or neck problems

Please do not attempt if you are pregnant

The next two movements, Pose of Tranquillity in the Lotus Position and the Pose of a Fish in the Lotus Position, are honestly a dream come true and well worth working at. In the Lotus position you will gain amazing flexibility in your ankles, knees and hips, all the benefits of a long stay in the Shoulderstand are included and the movement is so relaxing. The facial muscles are soothed and the skin benefits tremendously from this movement. The Fish in the Lotus position tones the inner thigh area, expands the chest (so is most beneficial to asthma sufferers), corrects poor posture, tones the throat and jaw and makes you feel as though you have had a shoulder massage.

To do this movement, ability to do a good Lotus position is essential.

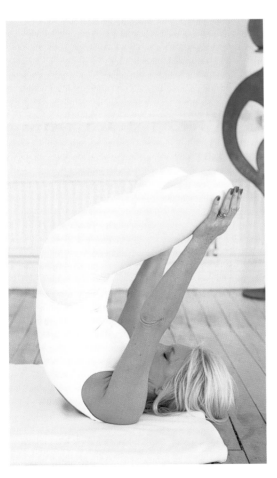

- Sit on your mat in the Full Lotus position (page 128). Now, retaining this position, lie down and gently lift your lower body from the floor.
- Support your back with your hands and stretch your legs upwards as far as possible. Only when you feel you can hold this position with ease, bring your arms up in front of your body and place your knees (still in the Lotus position) on your upheld hands. This is quite a major balance, so don't worry if at first you tend to wobble. There is a point of balance that you will reach when the movement feels so calm and peaceful you could stay there for ever, so please persevere.
- On reaching your final position, stay there to begin with for a count of 10, but lengthen the hold by increasing by 30 seconds per week until you can hold your maximum position for about 3 minutes.

  Follow immediately with the Pose of a Fish in the Lotus Position.

7 Pose of a Fish in the Lotus Position

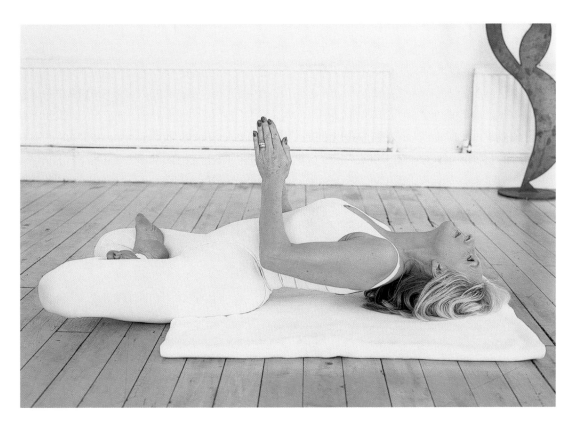

• To come out of the Pose of Tranquillity in the Lotus position, move your hands back to your waistline and very gently draw your knees towards your forehead, then gently roll down your back until your knees touch the floor. Place your hands under your buttocks, thumbs touching, and arch your back, bringing the top of your head onto the floor and, still keeping your legs locked in the Lotus position, place your hands in the prayer position on your chest.

• Relax in this position and take 3 slow, deep breaths, exhaling slowly after each one, then slowly and carefully place your hands by your sides, unwind your legs, stretch out your body and relax.

Beauty Tip

When you have mastered these two positions, use them often, especially when you feel tired or stressed. Before doing them, cleanse your skin; then, apply a lovely moisturizer, a little eye cream and some eye drops. Relax for 5 minutes. Afterwards you will look and feel refreshed, calm and revitalized.

8 The Wide-Angled Plough

We first practised the Plough on page 96, so I hope that you have enjoyed the movement and now are ready to progress to some new exciting movements. Proceed with caution, only attempting the movements in order and moving on only when the previous phase becomes easy for you.

This relieves tension in the lower back and encourages extra flexibility in the hips.

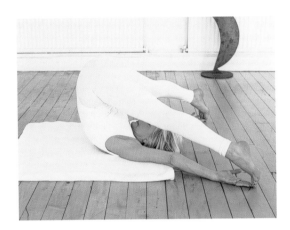

- Move into your maximum position of the Plough, then stay there and, if you are touching the floor with ease, then in your maximum position open your legs wide and stretch your hands out to your wide-open legs. Relax in your maximum position.

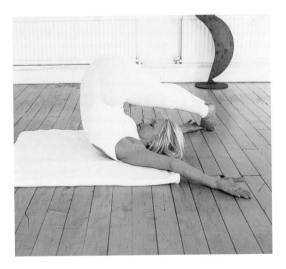

- When this is mastered with ease, take your right foot towards your left. Hold for a count of 3, then take your left foot towards your right one. This sounds easy, but your head, shoulders and arms must not move in this position – and again, going one way is often easier than the other. Once accomplished, move back into the Pose of a Plough, draw your knees to your forehead and then roll, vertebra by vertebra, slowly down until you are lying flat on the floor, then perform the pose of a Fish (see page 84).

LOOK 15 YEARS YOUNGER

9 The Noose

This increases the flexibility of your lower back, and tones and firms your buttocks.

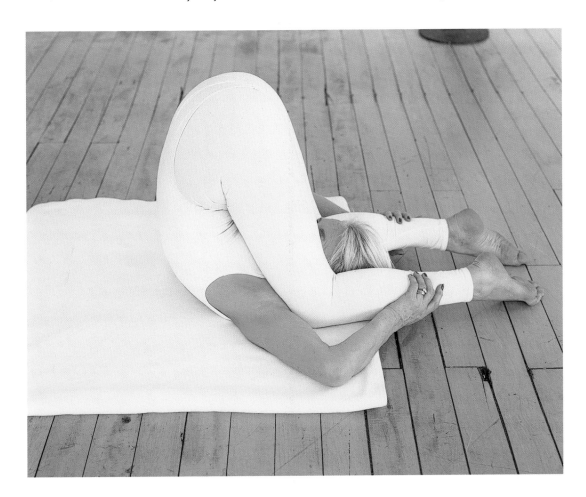

- In your maximum position in the Plough, gently lower your knees, aiming them near your ears. Place your hands on your calves and relax in this position, breathing normally and holding for a count of 10. Come out of the movement as in the previous exercise.

10 The Yoga Sleeping Pose

This movement increases the flexibility of your lower back, neck and shoulders and tones the kidneys, liver, spleen, gallbladder, intestines and bladder. It is also excellent for toning the spinal nerves. You are not going to believe this, but once you are in the full movement it really feels comfortable.

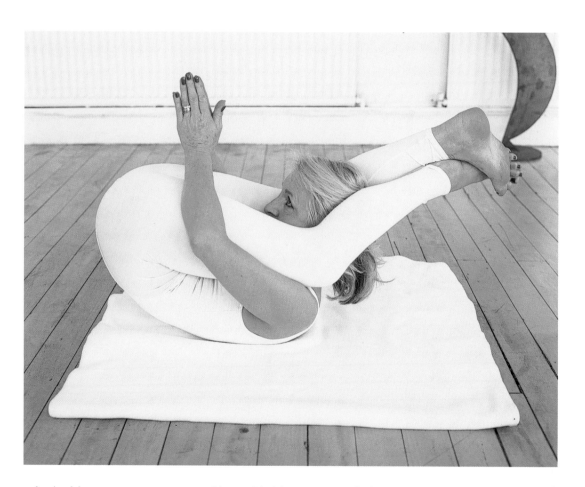

- In the Noose pose, cross your ankles and hold your calves and, carefully pushing your bottom slightly forwards, aim to lift your head between your knees. Please go carefully, this can take a while and don't strain. Once you have mastered the movement, hold for a count of 10 then uncross your ankles, draw your knees to your forehead and roll down your back one vertebra at a time and move into the Pose of a Fish (see page 84). Gently lie flat and relax your entire body. Well done!

11 The Classic Headstand

Well, I have saved the best till last. This movement is called 'the father of all yoga exercises' because of the intense rejuvenating effect it has on the entire body. It strengthens the lungs and circulation, and assists in aiding the flow of venous blood towards the heart. It benefits the skin and hair, refreshes the brain and helps the eyesight, hearing and memory.

The Headstand stimulates blood flow to the pituitary gland and the pineal body, so helping to keep these two glands in excellent condition.

The Headstand is an elixir of youth and, in my opinion, much better than a facelift, as it helps to prevent the adverse ageing effects of gravity.

This movement, although brilliant, needs to be done by a strong flexible body, which is why I have left it to the end. By now you should be feeling great, and I am so pleased that you have got this far. Now please do this movement carefully and don't try to rush it. In the first stages do it by a wall to prevent any fear of falling.

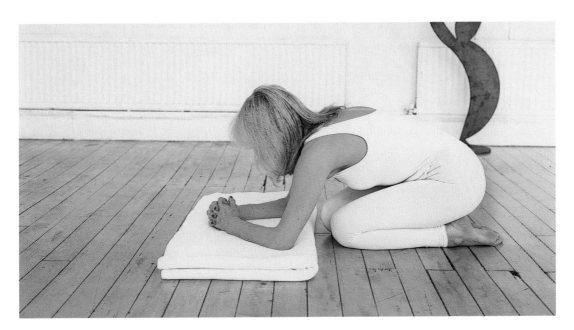

- Fold your blanket into a nice thick pad and place it on the floor by a wall. Interlock your hands together and place them on your mat. Now lift one hand up and ensure that it just touches the inside of the other elbow. This shows that your elbows are exactly the correct distance apart, so re-interlock your hands, keeping your elbows in this position.

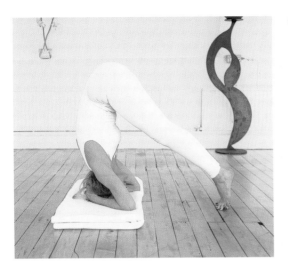

• Place your head on your mat so that it is framed by your interlocked hands. Lift your bottom in the air and walk your feet towards your head. When you have reached your maximum position, hold it for a count of 5, then kneel down and, keeping your head down, hold for a count of 10 to ensure your circulation returns to normal. Practise this position every day for 2-3 weeks before trying to progress further. By doing this you will accustom your head to the extra blood flow, and greatly strengthen your neck. All this is necessary preparation work for the Headstand.

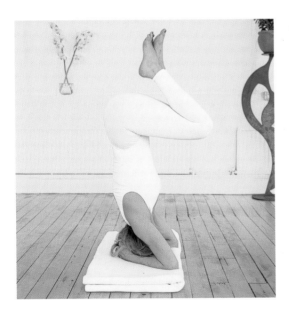

• When you have completed your preliminary stage, you will find your feet seem to want to leave the floor, so place your mat by the wall and move into your prepared position, then let your feet leave the floor as you come up into a crouching position.

On the first day he should remain only a little while in the headstand with legs in the air. This is viparitakarani, increase the practice time a little each day. After 6 months grey hairs and wrinkles disappear.

HATHA YOGA PRADIPIKA
CHAPTER 9 V80-82

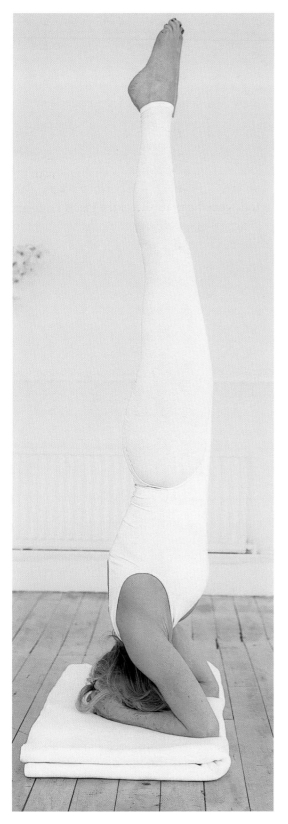

• Stay in this position to firmly establish your balance for a few seconds, then gently straighten your legs. Once in the maximum Headstand stay in it just for a few seconds to start with and increase the hold gradually until you are holding the position for about 2-3 minutes. To come out of the Headstand, bend your knees, move back into the crouching position and slowly lower yourself to the floor, keeping your legs together, then lower your bottom to your heels and relax. Keep your head down for a count of 10 to allow your circulation to return to normal, then slowly return to a kneeling position. Relax and well done!

12 Half-Split and Eagle in Headstand

When your Headstand becomes calm and steady, it's great to try to do some of the movements in this position. The Eagle is a great test of co-ordination and balance, and also wonderful for the flexibility and shape of your legs.

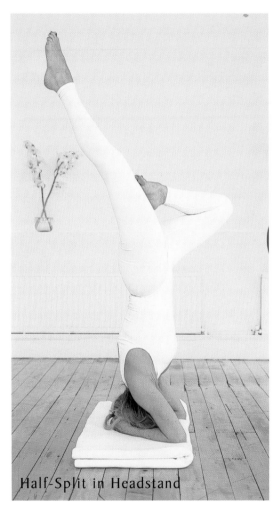

Half-Split in Headstand

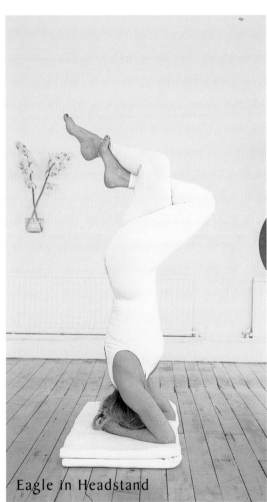

Eagle in Headstand

- In Full Headstand, carefully slide your right foot down your left thigh and hold for 5. Move back ino the Headstand and then repeat with the left leg.

- In Full Headstand, carefully take your left thigh over your right one and entwine your left calf around your right.
- Hold for a count of 5, then carefully unlock your legs and do the movement on the other side. Come down as for the classic Headstand.

LOOK 15 YEARS YOUNGER

Meditation

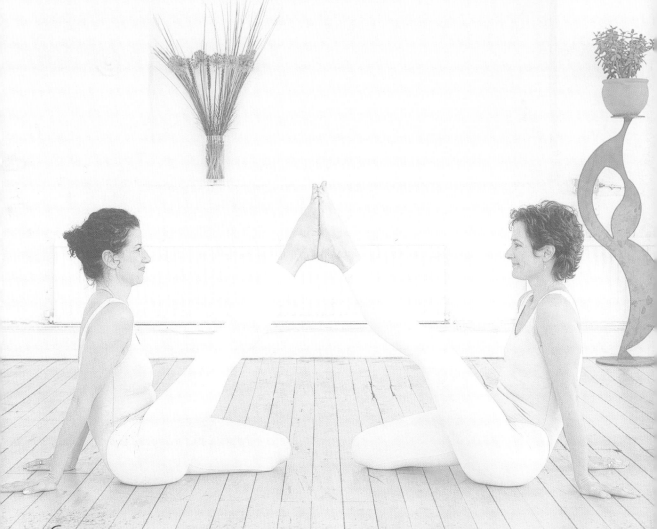

‛The mind in its own place and in itself can make a Heaven of Hell
and a Hell of Heaven.’

JOHN MILTON (1608–1674)

‛These days everybody wants Botox. I have had it myself only twice
– since the meditation I don't need it.’

JEYA PRAKASH, CONSULTANT PLASTIC SURGEON BASED IN HARLEY STREET

We have now fully discussed yoga's wonderful system of exercises, breathing, healthy eating and deep relaxation – all leading to a beautiful, youthful body, greater energy and a tremendous feeling of well-being.

Living in today's high-pressure world, however, can be exceedingly difficult: full of highs and lows, moments of tension, deep-seated anxiety, insecurity, frustration, struggle, noise and work overload, etc., all of which can lead to inner turmoil which can adversely effect both the body and mind. We try to sort ourselves out by resorting to the usual remedies – drinking strong coffee and other stimulants to give us more energy, alcohol to help us relax and sleeping pills to calm our overactive brains and help us to sleep. But these measures work only on the *symptoms* and not the *cause* of the problem. The cause is our inability to still our brain and make it calm and serene, and the overload of stimuli can result in chronic stress that can eventually lead to disease.

The amazing thing is that well over 5,000 years ago the yogis of ancient India realized that by learning to calm the mind we can help ourselves to a feeling of calm and peace, and by so doing alleviate the damaging effects of stress on the body and mind. Calming the mind, however, is difficult, and like the yoga exercises quite simply gets better with practice. There are many techniques, collectively referred to as *meditation*. Because we are all different, it is vital to find the method that works best for you.

How to Meditate

Sit in a comfortable position with your back straight. The Lotus position is ideal, but by no means essential. If you are not yet comfortable in it, then a crossed-leg position, kneeling position or your favourite armchair will do fine.

Make sure that you are warm enough, as your temperature can drop a little during meditation. Make sure that you will not be disturbed. If you have an appointment later, it is wise to set an alarm clock for your allocated meditation time, as it is not unusual to fall asleep during your first attempts at meditation.

o Now, close your eyes and concentrate on your breathing. Don't try to change it or regulate it, just bring your attention to it.
o If your mind wanders – and it does even for experienced meditators – just bring your attention back to your breathing. Please don't think that you are 'bad' at meditating if your mind wanders, just relax and gently bring your mind back to your breathing and allow all other thoughts to just slip away.

The above technique is my preferred method of meditation. Other ways include focusing on a special object like a beautiful flower or leaf, a special piece of crystal or rock, a candle flame (make sure that it is in a safe place if you think you might fall asleep), a religious symbol or literally any single object that works for you is fine.

Some people prefer to repeat a *mantra*. Choose a word like 'peace' or 'calm', or the yoga word *om* (pronounced 'aum'). This word is sacred to yoga and means 'what was, what is and what shall be.' Take a deep breath in and, as you exhale, say it softly and slowly, making your exhalation and the sound last as long as possible, then repeat it over and over again until a feeling of peace flows through you.

Start with 10 minutes of meditation, gradually increasing to 20 minutes. Do your meditation at a time to suit your own schedule. Early morning is traditionally a good time for meditation, but if your house is in chaos then just choose a time when you can relax and enjoy the peace and calm it will give you.

When the mind is busy and frequently overloaded with worries about the past and anxieties about the future, the brain in this state emits rapid beta brain waves. Once we start to calm the mind and focus on one object or our breathing, the mind stays in the present tense, which is free from stressful thoughts. When this feeling of calm and peace flows through our being the brain starts to emit slower and more rhythmic alpha brain waves. This lovely, peaceful sense of calm pervades our whole being, breathing slows down and stress hormone levels and blood pressure fall. Meditators find that they are less prone to stress and depression; they also have more energy, need less sleep and look younger and more radiant then non-meditators.

Don't Expect Instant Results

One of the problems of meditation for Westerners is that nothing much happens at first. You find it difficult to switch off and wonder if it is doing you any good. Please persevere, mediation does require practice and you will benefit from all your meditations. Eventually you will feel very clear, calm and focused, and frequently you will receive new, clear insights into a particular area of your life, and problems will seem easier to solve. Please don't grudge the time taken for meditation, as you are always more productive and proactive after meditation than before.

By meditating we are not trying to find peace and calm, they are already within us; we are trying to get rid of the incredible overload of mental stimuli to enable us to give our natural peace a place in our hectic lives.

Once you have been meditating for a while you may experience a beautiful relaxed and thought-free feeling – this is known as 'going into the gap'. As you continue to meditate, this will become more frequent. Here you experience contact with the universal spirit, which allows access to unlimited intelligence. You then stop relying on the opinion of others and become guided from within. You realize that you manifest your own destiny and experience a beautiful inner joy and confidence, and nothing is impossible for you. Things don't seem to worry you as much; you learn to trust your own gut instincts – which, of course, are the real you – and frequently, when your mind is calm, new ideas and solutions to problems just arrive out of the blue. All this results in a lovely feeling of deep inner peace and self-confidence.

Things will still go wrong; the cleaners will still ruin your best suit; you will still get held up in traffic, etc., and the problems of daily life will not go away, but deep down inside you won't worry as much because you will have learned to accept these things as part of life. You stay calm and focused on your goals, and regard the hassles of life as almost necessary hurdles and challenges on life's amazing journey, so that no matter what happens you can still look at a beautiful flower or tree and just be happy in spite of it all.

You do not need to leave your room, remain sitting at your table and listen. Do not even listen, simply wait. Do not even wait be quiet, still and solitary. The world will freely offer itself to you to be unmasked, it has no choice. It will roll in ecstasy at your feet.

FRANZ KAFKA

On a purely cosmetic basis, there is simply nothing that will erase your lines and wrinkles more than meditation – again I quote from the respected leading Consultant Cosmetic Plastic Surgeon, Jeya Prakash:

At home I practise meditation for 20 minutes every day. After 5 minutes of my mantra, the stress goes out of my head and I have a few minutes of completely static pure mind. Meditation is like washing your body from the inside. I follow it with 10 minutes of yoga. People say I look fresher, more vibrant. This is the real secret of youthful skin.

JEYA PRAKASH

I totally agree. Your face is a reflection of how you are inside. If you want to get rid of a sagging tense face – cleanse, tone and nourish from within.

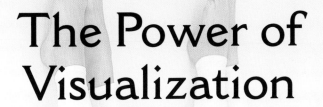

The Power of Visualization

If one advances confidently in the direction of his dreams, and endeavours to live the life which he has imagined he will meet with a success unexpected in common hours.

HENRY DAVID THOREAU

Once the mind is quiet and calmed by deep breathing, yoga exercises and meditation, we can then learn to control the mind and discipline it to create and enjoy our heart's desire. This power is not unusual – we are in fact using it every moment of every day. It is the power of our *imagination*. Yoga teaches us how to take control and use this incredible power to our own advantage.

In this way we can learn to create a fabulous life and a fantastic future, and fill our lives with health, happiness, hope and creativity instead of lack, fear, limitations, worry and difficulties.

We are creating our own lives by the thoughts we habitually think. When we imagine something, we create an idea or mental picture or a sense of something. By learning to discipline our minds we can learn to create for ourselves in our own minds a very clear picture of what we would like to manifest in our lives. Now, by stilling our minds and concentrating on that image at least three times a day, we start to make the image appear very real in our lives.

As we concentrate on the end product we start to get excited about our image – this gives it more positive creative energy until the thing we have pictured is achieved.

This power can be used to create anything in your life, from better health or a better body to a new job, better relationships or more money. It can also help you correct a habit such as smoking or drinking too much.

Let's take a small practical example. Say your living room needs to be decorated – it's dark and gloomy and you would like it to look fresh and bright.

1. First formulate in your mind exactly how you would like it to look. If you don't have a clear idea, find some interior design magazines, flick through these and choose several images that will help you to choose a scheme for your room. Don't think about lack of money, the size of your room, how there are no decent curtain-makers in the area, etc. Think instead of how you would really like it to look.
2. Now draw a floor plan of the new furniture arrangement.
3. Explore the shops for the colours you would like to use, and ask for samples of fabrics, paints, flooring, etc.
4. Make a sample board so you can see how your colours and fabrics relate to each other both in daylight and artificial light.
5. Now, three times a day, go into a quiet meditative state and then visualize your room transformed to your liking.
6. Eventually your mind accepts this picture as how the room *is*.
7. Now, with this firmly fixed plan in mind, start putting your ideas into action. Maybe at first just paint the walls, if time and money are limited in the beginning.

8. You must, however, keep visualizing the finished room three times a day, otherwise it is easy to give up or to allow other things to divert your attention.
9. By keeping your plan in mind when you are out shopping, your mind will focus on things to help you complete it. Maybe one day you will see the perfect vase, or a friend will recommend someone to make curtains and cushions for you within your budget, etc.
10. As you keep focusing on the finished product, more and more things and people will come to your aid, and eventually your beautiful room will be a reality.

Now, you might say that there is nothing unusual about the above example. I agree! There isn't, and if the above formula were applied to every room in your house, you would then have the house of your dreams.

By applying this formula to different aspects of your life, you can create the life of your dreams.

So what normally happens is that we get caught up, difficulties bog us down, etc. Let's take that room again and illustrate a relatively normal response. The living room needs decorating, so you look through the magazine and:

o You think 'how beautiful' – but it's out of your budget;
o You haven't got time for the planning;
o You put it off for a bit;
o   You do plan the room, but can't think when to start, so the plan goes in a drawer somewhere;
o You paint the walls and it looks a bit better, so the room will do for a bit;
o You go for coffee with a friend and discuss how difficult it is to find good workmen these days, etc.

The list is endless. This is what normally happens. But when you learn to quieten the mind and focus on your goal at least *three times a day* every day, you will find the plan is permanently in your mind and, regardless of limitations, money, time, difficulties, *it will be achieved*.

When you are inspired by some great purpose, some extraordinary project, all your thoughts break their bonds, your mind transcends limitation, your consciousness expands in every direction and you find yourself in a new, great and wonderful world. Dormant forces, faculties and talents become alive and you discover yourself to be a greater person by far than you have ever imagined yourself to be.

PATANJALI, YOGA SUTRAS

How Power Visualization Works

Our master teachers through the ages have always known that our thoughts determine our destiny.

Ask and it will be given to you, seek and you will find, knock and it will be opened unto you.

MATTHEW 7.7

If thou canst believe, all things are possible to him that believeth.

MARK 9.23

What we vividly imagine, ardently desire, enthusiastically act upon, must inevitably come to pass.

COLIN P SISSON

The greatest discovery of my generation is that human beings can alter their lives by altering their attitudes of mind.

WILLIAM JAMES

Your mind will be like its habitual thoughts, for the soul becomes dyed with the colour of its thoughts.

MARCUS AURELIUS 5.16

I am responsible for what I see, I choose the feelings I experience and I decide upon the goal that I would achieve and everything that seems to happen to me I ask for and receive as I have asked.

A COURSE IN MIRACLES

Nowadays our scientific experts seek to explain this by teaching us that we are all, along with everything else in the universe, composed of a force or energy and are all part of one huge vibrating energy field. As human beings we are extremely fortunate to be equipped with an incredible nervous system and thought processes enabling us to make changes in our lives simply by changing the thoughts we think. Thoughts are also energy vibrations that are magnetic and attract and create things in our lives. By changing our thoughts, and thereby changing our energy field, we can create changes in the wider energy field and so can start to make positive changes in our own lives and, eventually, manifest our own destiny. These changes can be brought about by the power of thought. Putting it simply, whatever you put your attention and intention on will grow stronger in your life, and whatever you take your attention and intention off will grow weaker and gradually disappear.

Inherent in every intention and desire is the mechanics for its fulfilment. Intention and desire in the field of pure potentiality have infinite organizing power. And when we increase an intention in the fertile ground of pure potentiality we put this infinite organizing power to work for us.

DEEPAK CHOPRA

We can now see how yoga (the union between body, mind and spirit) works so well for us. By creating an excellent healthy body with your yoga exercises, energizing and calming the mind with deep breathing, increasing the power of concentration and focus by performing the balances and learning one-point focus and calm in meditation, our minds are perfectly equipped for us to put our clear desires into the energy field.

This brilliant technique can be used to create anything we desire, from better health to a new job, more money to better relationships. I know it all sounds just too simple and your logical brain comes back with at least 50 reasons of why it won't work:

o   There are no decent jobs out there.
o   You can't afford to do the job you like because you have three kids and a mortgage
o   You have always had bad health.
o   Bad luck runs in your family.
o   There is no way you can earn extra money; you are just no good at anything.
o   You come home tired as it is, and will just have to get by with the salary you have.
o   Every relationship you have had goes sour.
o   You just seem to pick the wrong people.
o   At school they said you were only average and would never amount to anything.
o   You don't have the right contacts.
o   It's whom you know that makes the difference.

The list just goes on and on, and these are just a few of the obstacles that most people think of as soon as a desire comes into their mind. The great thinkers of this world, however, have always thought of the *outcome* of their desires, and not the hurdles along their path.

Once you start thinking in this way and putting your desires in a clear concise way, writing them down and putting them into your thoughts at least three times a day with calm serenity and total belief in the outcome, you will find that your dreams are fulfilled with effortless ease.

If you have faith as a grain of mustard seed, nothing shall be impossible unto you.

MATTHEW 7.20

But if your mind constantly thinks about the worries, troubles and obstacles in your path of life, then these will manifest in your life.

The thing which I greatly feared is come upon me, and that which I was afraid of is come unto me.

JOB 3.25

Once we learn this amazing power of the human mind and refuse to think of the obstacles in our path, we can then focus on our goals with calm, peace and serenity, knowing that the things we desire will manifest in our lives.

Whosoever shall say unto this mountain, 'be thou removed, and be thou cast into the sea' and shall not doubt in his heart, but shall believe that these things which he saith shall come to pass, he shall have whatsoever he saith.

MARK 11.23

The last quote, I believe, is one of the most powerful quotes of all time. Our mountains are our troubles, difficulties, sense of inferiority and negative thought patterns. Once you believe that your mountains or difficulties can be overcome, and focus on the outcome or goal of your dreams, your life *can* change.

How to Use This Wonderful Power

First, decide what you would like. This might sound crazy, but most people will say with a grin, 'Oh, I don't know … a better life or more money, etc.' You must be *specific*. Say, for example, you wanted to drive your car from London to Inverness. You would need a road map, a car in good condition, probably a place to stay en route to break your journey, adequate money for your petrol and food for the journey, and sufficient time to complete the journey. This is just simple planning, but without it you won't get there.

Now your life is your journey, and you must be specific.

o   Where do you want to go?
o   What do you want to achieve?
o   Where do you want to live?
o   How do you want to look?
o   How healthy and fit do you want to be?
o   How much money do you want to earn?
o   What places would you like to visit?
o   What car would you like to drive?
o   What job would you like to have?
o   What would be the house of your dreams?
o   How many children would you like to have?
o   What hobbies would you like to take up?

If you have never answered these questions before, sit down in a quiet place for about half an hour and just answer each one honestly and calmly without limits. Make sure you do this regardless of your age, present position, etc.

Now you have your road maps.

1. Now, put the five most important goals on a card in a brief form in the *present* tense, for example: 'I am a very fit and healthy architect earning £200,000 per year. I live in a beautiful old house in the country with my wife and two children.' Make sure that the picture you have described represents your ideal picture of your ideal life.
2. Carry this card with you and look at it at least three times a day – on waking (before your meditation), at lunch, and before bed.
3. By doing this you will start *being* the architect and your dream life will start to become a reality. Every day, make sure you do something to help you achieve your goals.
4. Meanwhile, don't make your happiness in life dependent on the fulfilment of every part of your dream. Simply decide now to be happy, no matter what, and to enjoy every part of your journey towards your dream.
5. Believe that your dreams will be manifested, expect hurdles and challenges along the way and be flexible. Sometimes on the way to a dream, something better turns up. Just believe that the great goodness that surrounds you has wonderful plans for you, sometimes better than your dreams.

Thou shall decree a thing and it shall be established unto thee. And the light shall shine upon thy ways.

JOB 22.28

In this way your dreams will gradually be fulfilled, easily and effortlessly. Your subconscious mind will guide you, new ideas will start to flow, the roadblocks on the way to your dreams will gradually be overcome and you will start to live the life that once was only in your dreams.

Mind is the master power that moulds and makes.
And we are mind and evermore we take the tool of thought and shaping what we will
Bring forth a thousand joys or a thousand ills.
We think in secret and it comes to pass
Our world is but our looking glass.

JAMES ALLEN, AUTHOR OF *AS A MAN THINKETH*

My 30 Tips for Looking and Feeling Young For Ever

1. Start every day with 15 minutes of yoga.

2. Drink 8 glasses of water per day

3. Eat fresh fruit, fresh vegetables, whole grains, nuts and seeds, chicken, fish and a little cheese, natural organic yoghurt and olive oil and cut out all junk foods.

4. Correct your posture – good posture instantly makes you look 10 years younger.

5. Calm and cool stress always with 10 slow, deep breaths, exhaling slowly after each one – stress is ageing.

6. Count your blessings – an attitude of gratitude is beautiful.

7. Clear out your clutter – this releases energy and allows new things to come into your life.

8. Meditate daily, it will get rid of the 21st-century worry-hurry sickness which can cause chronic stress, pale skin, dull hair and a tense and pinched look. Meditation gives you calm, peace, radiance and energy.

9. Sleep well – your body repairs itself during sleep.

10. Sleep flat – that is, without a pillow. You'll have to do this very gradually, especially if you sleep on a pile of pillows to start with, but as your posture improves by day, it will improve by night by sleeping flat. Sleeping flat helps get rid of a double chin and can allow extra oxygen to the brain during sleep, so making you feel great on waking.

11. Laugh often – it does you and your body a world of good, and is a great stress-buster.

12. Keep making new goals – it's great to be planning and achieving regardless of age, and it is exciting.

13. Have fresh flowers in your house or flat always. They do wonders for you – if you are broke, then choose one beautiful flower and enjoy it.

14. Stop moaning – it is ageing, very ageing.

15. Always keep interested in people, your hobbies, your work, your friends.

16. Keep optimistic, no matter what.

17. If you want to lose weight, eat less, keep busy, keep out of the kitchen, eat slowly and never between meals, and never eat standing up.

18. Love yourself – none of us is perfect, but it is vital to just love yourself for what you are. You really are lovely.

19. Do a good turn each day.

20. Make a 'to do' list every day. Enumerate things in order of importance, then start at number 1 and work through the list calmly and slowly. Then, even if you only do the first six things, you'll have at least accomplished your priorities.

21. Keep a 'good time book' – making a note of all your good times. It makes a great read on blue days.

22. Love life in all its forms, love your friends, love your job, love your cat. Just simply love life – it is great to be alive in this fascinating, wonderful world.

23. Forgive everyone immediately. Holding grudges will damage you much more than them as it will block your energy centres.

24. Trust your own gut feelings – they are the real you.

25. Enjoy fresh air. A daily walk in the fresh air does wonders and will give you a healthy glow.

26. Have your teeth cleaned and whitened by your dentist. This will make you look much younger and brighter.

27. Get a good, easy-to-manage hairdo and avoid the stiff-set look.

28. Dry skin brush every day before your bath or shower to stimulate your circulation.

29. Enjoy a light tan – I have never liked the vampire look and, of course, you must use adequate sun protection, but I do believe a little sun does wonders for both your mind and body.

30. Put your feet up, be good to yourself and give yourself a pat on the back or a little present as soon as you achieve a goal – you deserve it!

Thank you for staying with me to the end, I do hope this book has helped you.

My promise was to make you look and feel 15 years younger in 15 minutes a day. In the beginning chapter we discussed what was meant by ageing. I do hope I have shown you the way to a beautiful, flexible, firm and toned body, beautiful skin, glossy hair, great shape, radiant health and well-being, inner calm, energy and the power to achieve anything your heart desires – in fact, all the attributes of youth.

Yoga has helped me so much, and I do hope it helps you. Please let me know how you get on by writing to me care of my publisher.

With my love
Barbara Currie

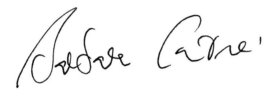

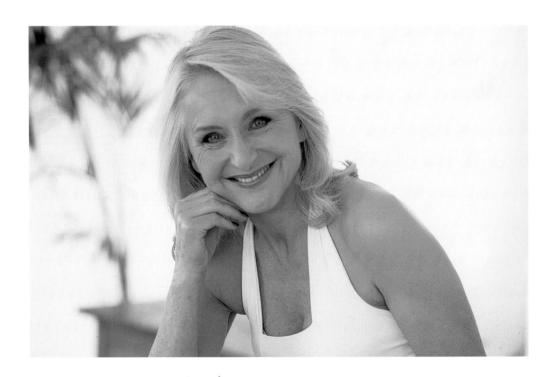